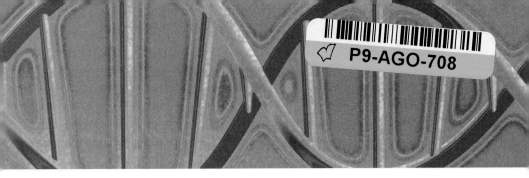

Psychopathology
in the
Genome and
Neuroscience Era

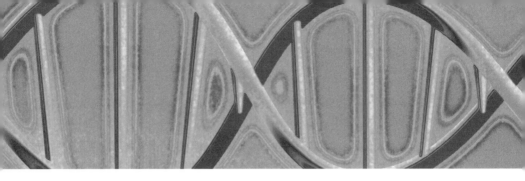

Psychopathology in the Genome and Neuroscience Era

Edited by

Charles F. Zorumski, M.D.
Eugene H. Rubin, M.D., Ph.D.

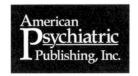

American Psychiatric Publishing, Inc.

Washington, DC
London, England

Copyright © 2005 American Psychiatric Publishing, Inc.
ALL RIGHTS RESERVED

Manufactured in the United States of America on acid-free paper
09 08 07 06 05   5 4 3 2 1
First Edition

Typeset in Adobe's Palatino and Helvetica Neue

American Psychiatric Publishing, Inc.
1000 Wilson Boulevard
Arlington, VA 22209-3901
www.appi.org

Library of Congress Cataloging-in-Publication Data
Psychopathology in the genome and neuroscience era / edited by Charles F. Zorumski, Eugene H. Rubin.—1st ed.
    p. ; cm.
  Includes bibliographical references and index.
  ISBN 1-58562-242-7 (pbk. : alk. paper)
  1. Mental illness—Genetic aspects. 2. Psychology, Pathological—Etiology.
  [DNLM: 1. Mental Disorders—genetics. WM 140 P9763 2005] I. Zorumski, Charles F. II. Rubin, Eugene H.
  RC455.4.G4P79 2005
  616.8'0442—dc22

                                                              2005011186

British Library Cataloguing in Publication Data
A CIP record is available from the British Library.

Contents

PART I

The Future of Psychiatric Genetics

PART II

Diagnosis and Prevention of Psychiatric Disorders

PART III

Neurobiology and Psychiatric Disorders

PART IV

The Future of Psychiatric Education

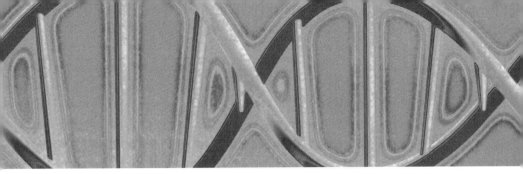

Contributors

John N. Constantino, M.D.
Departments of Psychiatry and Pediatrics, Division of Child and Adolescent Psychiatry, Washington University School of Medicine, St. Louis, Missouri

Linda B. Cottler, Ph.D.
Professor, Epidemiology and Prevention Research Group, Department of Psychiatry, Washington University School of Medicine, St. Louis, Missouri

Wayne C. Drevets, M.D.
Chief, Section on Neuroimaging in Mood and Anxiety Disorders, Mood and Anxiety Disorders Program, National Institute of Mental Health, Bethesda, Maryland

Anne E. Farmer, M.D.
MRC Social, Genetic and Developmental Psychiatry Centre, Institute of Psychiatry, King's College London

Elliot S. Gershon, M.D.
Foundation Funds Professor of Psychiatry and Human Genetics, Department of Psychiatry, University of Chicago, Chicago, Illinois

Alison M. Goate, D.Phil.
Departments of Psychiatry, Genetics, and Neurology, Washington University School of Medicine, St. Louis, Missouri

James J. Hudziak, M.D.
Professor of Psychiatry and Medicine, Director of Child Psychiatry and Behavioral Genetics, Center for Youth, Children, and Families, University of Vermont College of Medicine, Burlington, Vermont

Peter McGuffin, M.B., Ph.D.
MRC Social, Genetic and Developmental Psychiatry Centre, Institute of Psychiatry, King's College London

Kathleen R. Merikangas, Ph.D.
Senior Investigator, National Institute of Mental Health, National Institutes of Health, Department of Health and Human Services, Bethesda, Maryland

William E. Narrow, M.D., M.P.H.
Division of Research, American Psychiatric Association, Arlington, Virginia

Rosalind J. Neuman, Ph.D.
Departments of Psychiatry and Genetics, Division of Child and Adolescent Psychiatry, Washington University School of Medicine, St. Louis, Missouri

Petra Nowotny, Ph.D.
Department of Psychiatry, Washington University School of Medicine, St. Louis, Missouri

John W. Olney, M.D.
John P. Ferghner Professor of Neuropsychopharmacology, Department of Psychiatry, Washington University School of Medicine, St. Louis, Missouri

Donald S. Rae, M.S.
Division of Research, American Psychiatric Association, Arlington, Virginia

Darrel A. Regier, M.D., M.P.H.
Director, Division of Research, American Psychiatric Association, Arlington, Virginia

Eugene H. Rubin, M.D., Ph.D.
Professor of Psychiatry, Vice Chair for Education, Department of Psychiatry, Washington University School of Medicine, St. Louis, Missouri

Maritza Rubio-Stipec, D.Sc.
Division of Research, American Psychiatric Association, Arlington, Virginia

Scott Smemo, B.A.
Department of Psychiatry, Washington University School of Medicine, St. Louis, Missouri

Richard D. Todd, Ph.D., M.D.
Departments of Psychiatry and Genetics, Division of Child and Adolescent Psychiatry, Washington University School of Medicine, St. Louis, Missouri

Charles F. Zorumski, M.D.
Samuel B. Guze Professor and Head, Department of Psychiatry, Washington University School of Medicine, St. Louis, Missouri

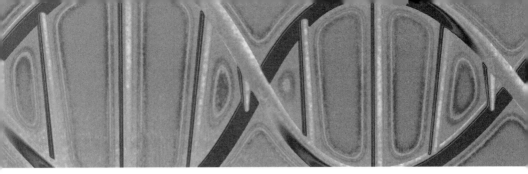

Preface

Recent advances in genetics and neuroscience promise to enhance our understanding of human behavior and psychopathology. How the field incorporates the coming avalanche of information will influence not only how mental health professionals diagnose and treat patients, but also how the next generation of professionals is trained. The goal of the 2003 annual meeting of the American Psychopathological Association was to examine several specific areas in which advances in genetics and neuroscience are likely to influence psychopathology research and education in the near future. These areas include understanding the influence of genetics on the diagnosis and prevention of psychiatric disorders and understanding the role of neurodevelopment and neurodegeneration in psychopathological processes.

Charles F. Zorumski, M.D.
Eugene H. Rubin, M.D., Ph.D.

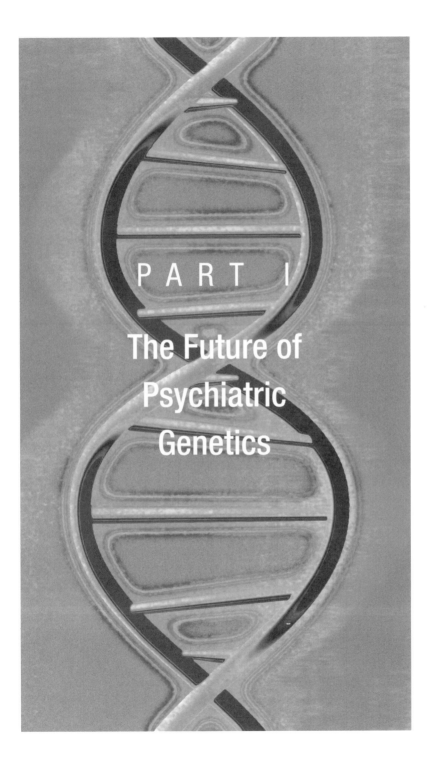

PART I

The Future of
Psychiatric
Genetics

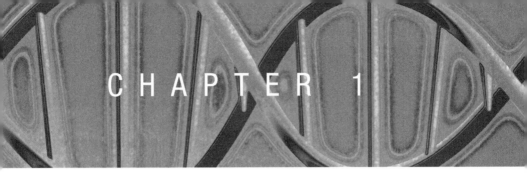

CHAPTER 1

Bridging Genetics and Epidemiology of Mental Disorders

Kathleen R. Merikangas, Ph.D.

The past decade has witnessed dramatic advances in knowledge regarding the genetic basis of numerous human diseases, including various cancers, cystic fibrosis, and neurological diseases such as Huntington's disease, neurofibromatosis, and Alzheimer's disease. As the Human Genome Project has reached its fruition, there has been tremendous enthusiasm for the possible implications for etiology, treatment, and prevention of human disease as well as for increased understanding of normal human biology. However, this progress has not yet been fully realized for most complex human disorders (i.e., disorders with high population prevalence [>1%], indistinct boundaries between affected and unaffected status, and non-Mendelian patterns of familial aggregation). Although there have been developments that now hold promise

This chapter is adapted in part from Merikangas KR, Risch N: "Will the Genomics Revolution Revolutionize Psychiatry?" *American Journal of Psychiatry* 160: 625–635, 2003; and Merikangas KR: "Genetic Epidemiology: Bringing Genetics to the Population—the NAPE Lecture 2001." *Acta Psychiatrica Scandinavica* 105: 3–13, 2002. Used with permission.

for identifying genes underlying some of the major mental disorders, genetic risk factors for the majority of mental disorders have not yet been established.

In this chapter, I describe the importance of a conceptual shift from identifying major genes for mental disorders to understanding which genes—in which contexts (both biological and environmental)—confer susceptibility to or protection from mental disorders.

EVIDENCE FOR GENES INVOLVED IN MENTAL DISORDERS

There are several comprehensive reviews of the evidence from family, twin, and adoption studies regarding the role of genetic factors in the etiology of mental disorders. Ironically, genetic epidemiologic approaches have been applied far more to mental disorders than to any other class of human diseases. The evidence for the influence of genes in controlled or population-based studies has been reviewed by Merikangas and Swendsen (1997). Table 1–1 presents an updated summary of the average risk ratios derived from studies of major mental disorders. The familial recurrence risks are significantly elevated for all of the major mental disorders, irrespective of the sampling and methods employed. The risk ratios are greatest for bipolar disorder and schizophrenia (ranging from 6 to 10); intermediate for substance dependence (averaging 4–8) and subtypes of anxiety, particularly panic (i.e., 5%); and lowest for major depression (averaging 2–3).

Evidence that linkage strategies lacked sufficient power for diseases with lower genotypic relative risks led to a shift, in the 1990s, to genomic association studies (Risch and Merikangas 1996). However, this approach requires a priori knowledge of the actual gene or genes involved prior to performing the test of the association; such knowledge is necessary to avoid the high false-positive rate attributable to the low prior probability that the polymorphisms examined in association studies are causally related to the diseases under study (Risch 2000). The same impediments that limited the success of linkage studies, including phenotypic heterogeneity, etiological heterogeneity, and low genotypic attributable risk, have also continued to plague association studies.

The major problems in defining future strategies for identifying genes for mental disorders are the lack of consistent findings from existing studies and the uncertainty regarding appropriate designs and methods for detecting genes for complex disorders. Replication of findings of association and linkage studies has been difficult not only for mental disorders but for all complex diseases. In a summary of linkage findings for

TABLE 1–1. Risk of major mental disorders among relatives in controlled family, twin, and adoption studies

Disorder	Family	Twin	Adoption
Bipolar disorder	5.5	0.6	9.2
Anxiety disorders	9.4	2.4	–
Major depression	6.8	2.4	1.8
Schizophrenia	8.9	4.4	4.3
Substance use disorders	4.5	6.3	2.1

6 of 32 complex diseases with the largest samples (i.e., asthma, bipolar affective disorder, psoriasis, schizophrenia, type 1 diabetes, and type 2 diabetes), only 2 of 52 studies confirmed linkage (i.e., type 1 diabetes and psoriasis). Increased success in the replication of linkage studies was associated with two study features: an increase in the sample size and ethnically homogeneous samples (Altmuller et al. 2001). Similar conclusions have been drawn regarding association studies of complex diseases. In a review of 600 positive genetic association studies, despite 166 diseases being studied three or more times, only 6 were found to be replicated consistently (Hirschhorn et al. 2002).

Resolution of the discrepancies in linkage findings is becoming increasingly important with the rapid advances in genomics. Exploration of explanations for discrepancies at the level of the phenotype definition, characterization of DNA markers, or statistical methods may provide a stronger base for a priori testing of particular candidate regions in future studies. One of the lessons learned from other diseases is the success achieved by integration of efforts to identify genes. A recent example of a successful initiative to promote collaboration among investigators involved in study of families with Crohn's disease yielded a successful identification of linkage even though the individual studies yielded inconclusive results (Cavanaugh and the IBD International Genetics Consortium 2001). Levinson et al. (1999) have developed a similar collaborative endeavor for genetic studies of schizophrenia that will provide a far more powerful approach than the small-scale, individual, investigator-based studies of the past.

SOURCES OF COMPLEXITY OF MENTAL DISORDERS

Two major issues concerning the complex patterns of inheritance with regard to psychiatric disorders are the lack of validity of the classification of psychiatric disorders (e.g., phenotypes, or observable aspects of diseases) and the complexity of the pathways from genotypes to psychiatric phenotypes (i.e., heterogeneity).

Lack of Validity of the Classification System

Psychiatric disorder phenotypes, based solely on clinical manifestations without pathognomonic markers, still lack conclusive evidence for the validity of classification and the reliability of measurement (Kendell 1989). This situation is not due to a lack of attention to classification in psychiatry; in fact, advances in the development of standardized classification and assessment methods have superseded those of most other clinically defined diagnostic entities. The development of structured interviews has enhanced comparability of diagnostic methods within the United States and worldwide. There is now an exciting venture designed to collect information on the prevalence of mental disorders, in which comparable diagnostic tools are being used in more than 20 countries under the auspices of World Mental Health 2000, sponsored by the World Health Organization (Kessler and Üstün 2000).

The results of epidemiological studies have illustrated the need for further development of the psychiatric diagnostic system (Kessler et al. 1994; Regier et al. 1990). The findings of inadequate coverage of care in current community and primary health care settings, the tendency for comorbidity to be more common than single disorders, and the lack of longitudinal stability of the major diagnostic categories have generated new research designed to examine the thresholds and boundaries of the major psychiatric disorders (e.g., Angst et al. 1997; Kessler et al. 1994). In his discussion of the validity of the psychiatric disorders, Kendell (1989) noted that it is unlikely that the etiological secrets of the major psychiatric disorders will be unlocked without accurate and valid identification of the syndromes themselves. Such validation has particular relevance in the search for biological markers, which depends in large part on the identification of discrete and homogeneous forms of disorder (Freedman et al. 1984).

The lack of pathognomonic signs for the major mental disorders has forced our continued reliance on the descriptive approach as the sole basis for diagnosis in psychiatry. The difficulty in classifying human cognition, behavior, and emotion is not unexpected in light of the complex psychological and physiological states underlying mental function, which are the product of the entire human experience in adaptation to the environment (Dolan 2002). Advances in the tools to detect human brain functioning in vivo have led to dramatic advances in knowledge about central nervous system function (McKhann 2002). However, this work is still in its infancy; future advances in neuroscience and behavioral science are likely to yield valuable information for understanding, and thus classifying, mental disorders.

Complex Patterns of Transmission

The application of advances in genomics to mental disorders is still limited by the complexity of the process through which genes exert their influence. There is substantial evidence that a lack of one-to-one correspondence between the genotype and phenotype exists for most of the major mental disorders. Phenomena such as *penetrance* (i.e., probability of phenotypic expression among individuals with susceptibility gene), *variable expressivity* (i.e., variation in clinical expression associated with a particular gene), *gene–environment interaction* (i.e., expression of genotype only in the presence of particular environmental exposures), *pleiotropy* (i.e., capacity of genes to manifest several different phenotypes simultaneously), *genetic heterogeneity* (i.e., different genes leading to indistinguishable phenotypes), and *polygenic* and *oligogenic modes of inheritance* (i.e., simultaneous contributions of multiple genes rather than effects based on Mendelian single-gene models) are characteristic of the mental disorders, as they are of numerous other complex disorders for which susceptibility genes have been identified (Gottesman and Shields 1972; Risch 1990). Other complicated situations include mitochondrial inheritance, imprinting, and epigenetic phenomena (Guttmacher and Collins 2002).

The high magnitude of comorbidity and co-aggregation of index disorders with other major psychiatric disorders (e.g., bipolar disorder and alcoholism, major depression and anxiety disorders, schizophrenia and drug dependence), in part an artifact of the classification system, has been demonstrated in both clinical and community studies (Galbaud du Fort et al. 1998; Maier and Merikangas 1996; Maier et al. 1995; Merikangas 1982; Merikangas et al. 1996, 1998). For example, alcoholism, a well-established complication of bipolar illness, may mask the underlying features of bipolarity, leading to phenotypic misclassification in genetic studies (Merikangas and Gelernter 1990). *Nonrandom mating* is also a common phenomenon in mental disorders that impedes evaluation of patterns of familial transmission (Merikangas 1982). *Assortative mating* is particularly pronounced for substance use disorders, in which substance dependence among spouses of substance-dependent probands may be as high as 90% (Merikangas 1982; Merikangas et al. 1992). These phenomena serve to increase the noise-to-signal ratio in defining the mental disorders for genetic studies. Studies that attempt to identify and disentangle the impact of these phenomena on phenotypic and endophenotypic expression in individuals and families will bring us closer to understanding the role of the underlying genes on the components of mental disorders.

FUTURE DIRECTIONS

Two areas of future research that are particularly promising for informing phenotypic validity include 1) genetic epidemiologic strategies and prospective longitudinal studies for phenotype refinement and 2) greater integration of genetics with basic neuroscience and behavioral sciences to elucidate potentially heritable components of psychiatric phenotypes.

Genetic Epidemiology: Moving Into the Community

In an editorial in *Science*, Peltonen and McKusick (2001) concluded that the best strategy for gene identification will ultimately be large epidemiological studies in diverse populations. The importance of epidemiology in the future of genetics has also been described by others, such as Risch (2000) and Khoury and Yang (1998), who predicted that population-based association studies will assume increasing importance in studying the role of genetic risk factors in complex human diseases. The concept of *heritability*, a purely statistical phenomenon, will be replaced by the concepts of relative risk to individuals and attributable risk in populations. Population-based epidemiological studies will be necessary to calculate the attributable, relative, and absolute risk of genetic risk factors identified in family-based linkage and association studies. Moreover, these authors anticipate that population-based case–control studies will have an increasing role in the genome-wide search for susceptibility genes for complex human disorders.

There is increasing interest in regenerating the field of genetic epidemiology, which can be distinguished from its parent disciplines in three specific ways: 1) its focus on population-based research, 2) its goal of detecting the joint effects of genes and environment, and 3) the incorporation of underlying biology of a disease into conceptual models (Thomas 2000). Unfortunately, the field of genetic epidemiology has become almost exclusively focused on statistical methods for identification of genes, as witnessed by recent trends in the journal *Genetic Epidemiology*.

As such, epidemiology has been detached from the field; in fact, the majority of scientists who perceive themselves as genetic epidemiologists have never had any formal training in epidemiology, because they often equate epidemiology solely with community-based sampling.

Five major applications of genetic epidemiology are needed to advance our understanding of mental disorders:

1. Establishment of population-based registries of mental disorders that will be increasingly valuable in validating the numerous genetic tests that will emerge from advances in human genetic research and the Human Genome Project (Yang et al. 2000)
2. Identification of more homogenous subtypes of mental disorders through family and high-risk group research investigating both biological and contextual factors
3. Investigation of familial patterns among affected and unaffected probands to estimate strength and mode of genetic transmission
4. Quantification of risk at the levels of the individual and population (i.e., absolute risk, relative risk, attributable risk)
5. Development of a richer conceptualization of environmental factors that may be important mediators of expression of genetic risk for mental disorders through integration of the tools of genetic epidemiology, behavioral neuroscience, developmental psychology, and neuroscience

The contributions of genetic epidemiology to the identification and translation of the public health significance of genes are summarized in Table 1–2.

Phenotypic Validation

Although genetic epidemiological study designs may provide a powerful source for validation of diagnostic criteria, such studies have not realized their full potential in psychiatry. The assumption that within-family similarity exceeds between-family similarity is critical to the role of genetics in testing the validity of nosology. These designs reduce the danger of genetic heterogeneity, which has been a major impediment to progress in psychiatric genetics. As described earlier, family and twin studies can be employed to study the validity of diagnostic categories by assessing core components of the phenotype, endophenotypes, or latent markers of disease risk; common versus distinct familial sources of comorbidity; and environmental exposures that potentiate or suppress gene expression.

TABLE 1–2.   Role of genetic epidemiology in the human genome era

Establish population-based norms for biological and genetic markers

Validate phenotypes

Quantify impact of genes on disease in individuals and general population

Identify environmental susceptibility and protective factors

Disseminate knowledge regarding meaning of susceptibility genes to general
  community

Inform development of guidelines for genetic testing and prenatal counseling

Prevent disease

Identification of Environmental Factors

It is ironic that psychiatry has recently focused far more on genes than on environmental factors that may be involved in the etiology of mental disorders. To date, no specific environmental etiological factors for mental disorders in general have been identified. Environmental research has focused on nonspecific life events, particularly those involving loss (in regard to mood disorders), impairments in parental and familial environment, and stress in general. However, none of these phenomena are specific to any of the mental disorders, and indeed they may be equally likely to affect individuals with other chronic diseases, such as cancer or heart disease. Future research designed to identify environmental factors that operate either specifically or nonspecifically on those with susceptibility to specific mental disorders may provide an important opportunity for prevention and intervention, once susceptibility genes have been identified. Increased knowledge of the developmental pathways of emotion, cognition, and behavior will expand our ability to identify specific environmental factors such as infection, poor diet, prenatal environment, and life experiences that mold the genetic architecture of mood regulation and cognition.

The importance of identifying environmental factors is illustrated by numerous examples of gene–environment interaction and genotype–phenotype correlations for diseases with known genetic bases. For example, the age at onset for Alzheimer's disease among carriers of the βAPP gene occurs later among those with the apolipoprotein E (*APOE*) ε2 allele and earlier among those with the *APOE* ε4 allele (St. George-Hyslop et al. 2000). The *BRCA1* gene for breast cancer is a tumor suppressor gene that tends to protect against cancer. An inherited mutation suppresses one copy of the gene, but some environmental event must occur to suppress the other copy. Radiation, low parity, and oral contraceptive use have been suggested as possible sources of somatic mutations (Whittemore 1999). Newman et al. (1997) credited the synergy between genetics and epidemiology in elucidating the initial gene findings, as well as subsequent identification of other susceptibility alleles and the environmental factors that may influence the risk of breast cancer in susceptible persons.

The malleability of environmental risk factors is a particularly important consideration in determining priorities for public health. Fixed factors such as sex, birth cohort, and ethnicity may be important in characterizing risk but cannot serve as targets of prevention. The major preventable environmental causes of death or illness are tobacco use, unhealthy diet, physical inactivity, excessive alcohol use, infections, trauma, and exposure to environmental toxins (Calabrese et al. 1997; Ishibe and Kelsey 1997).

Population-Based Studies

Population-based samples will be critical for translating findings emerging from the Human Genome Project for applications in public health and medicine (Khoury and Dorman 1998). Khoury et al. (2003) coined the term *human genome epidemiology* to denote the emerging field that uses systematic applications of epidemiological methods and approaches in population-based studies of the impact of human genetic variation on health and disease.

There are several reasons that population-based studies will be critical to the future of genetics. First, the prevalence of newly identified polymorphisms, whether single nucleotide polymorphisms or other variants, especially in particular population subgroups, is unknown. Second, current knowledge of genes as risk factors is based nearly exclusively on clinical and nonsystematic samples. Hence, the significance of the susceptibility alleles that have been identified for cancer, heart disease, diabetes, and so forth is unknown in the population at large. To provide accurate risk estimates, the next stage of research needs to move beyond samples identified through affected individuals to the population as a whole in order to obtain estimates of the risk of specific polymorphisms. Third, identification of risk profiles will require very large samples to assess the significance of vulnerability genes with relatively low expected population frequencies. Fourth, much as epidemiology can be used to quantify the risk associated with traditional disease risk factors, human genome epidemiology can be applied to provide information on the specificity, sensitivity, and impact of genetic tests to inform science and the individual (Yang et al. 2000).

Because genetic polymorphisms involved in complex diseases are likely to be nondeterministic (i.e., the marker predicts neither disease nor nondisease with certainty), traditional epidemiological risk factor designs can be used to estimate their impact (Ellsworth and Manolio 1999). As epidemiologists add genes to their risk equations, it is likely that the contradictory findings from studies that have generally employed solely environmental risk factors, such as diet, smoking, and alcohol use, will be resolved. Likewise, the studies that seek solely to identify genes will also continue to be inconsistent if they do not consider the effects of nongenetic biological parameters as well as environmental factors that contribute to the diseases of interest.

There are several types of risk estimates used in public health. The most common is *relative risk*, defined as the magnitude of the association between an exposure and disease. It is independent of the prevalence of the exposure. *Absolute risk* is the overall probability of developing a disease in an individual or in a particular population (Gordis 2000). *Attributable risk* is the difference between the risk of the disease in those exposed to a particular risk factor and the background risk of a disease in a population (i.e., the unexposed). *Population attributable risk* relates to the risk of a disease in a total population (exposed and unexposed) and indicates the amount the disease can be reduced in a population if an exposure is eliminated. Population attributable risk depends on the prevalence of the exposure or, in the case of genes, the gene frequency. *Genetic attributable risk* would indicate the proportion of a particular disease that would be eliminated if a particular gene or genes were not involved.

Role of Epidemiology in Translating Genomics to Public Health

The implications of genomics for public health have been widely discussed. However, it is clear that progress in genomics has far outweighed advances in our understanding of psychiatric phenotypes and the complexity underlying their etiology, and our current armamentarium for identifying genetic and environmental risk factors. Therefore, despite the extraordinary opportunity for elucidating disease pathogenesis afforded by the technical advances and availability of rapidly expanding genetic databases, their relevance to understanding, treating, or preventing major mental disorders has not been realized. It is likely that components of the mental disorders and their developmental expression will ultimately be mapped to specific brain systems and to

---

TABLE 1–3. Future trends in genetics of complex disorders

Collaboration will increase within the subdisciplines of genetics and among clinical, basic, and public health approaches to human disorders.

A search for "*the* gene" will be replaced by the search for "the genes" underlying many complex disorders.

Definition of biologically relevant phenotypes will reduce the uncertainty of clinical phenotypes.

Shift to forward-genetics approaches from current reverse-genetics approaches to complex diseases will lead to stronger integration of basic clinical science.

Descriptive genetic epidemiology will evolve into analytic genetic epidemiology.

Risk and protective environmental factors that may be informative for both etiology and prevention will be identified.

Population-based samples will be the major source of information on complex genetic diseases.

---

the genes that guide their development or disrupt their function.

Increased integration of advances in neuroscience (Hyman 2000) and genomics, along with information from nested case–control studies of population-based studies and longitudinal cohorts, innovations in our conceptualizations of the mental disorders, and the identification of specific risk and protective factors, will lead to more informed intervention strategies in psychiatry. As the role of genes as risk factors, rather than as the causes of human diseases, is elucidated, it will be essential to provide accurate risk estimation and to inform the public of the need for population-based integrated data on genetic, biological, and environmental risk factors. Table 1–3 summarizes future directions in the genetics of complex disorders (Merikangas et al. 2002).

The goal of genomics research is ultimately prevention, the cornerstone of public health. Integration of knowledge on genetic and other risk factors that confer susceptibility to developing mental disorders may ultimately provide an empirical basis for prevention of these widely disabling conditions. In the meanwhile, recurrence risk estimates from family studies constitute the best available knowledge from which to predict the risk of developing mental disorders.

REFERENCES

Altmuller J, Palmer LJ, Fischer G, et al: Genomewide scans of complex human diseases: true linkage is hard to find. Am J Hum Genet 69:936–950, 2001

Angst J, Merikangas KR, Preisig M: Subthreshold syndromes of depression and anxiety in the community. J Clin Psychiatry 58:6–10, 1997

Calabrese EJ, Stanek EJ, James RC, et al: Soil ingestion: a concern for acute toxicity in children. Environ Health Perspect 105:1354–1358, 1997

Cavanaugh J, IBD International Genetics Consortium: International collaboration provides convincing linkage replication in complex disease through analysis of a large pooled data set: Crohn disease and chromosome 16. Am J Hum Genet 68:1165–1171, 2001

Dolan RJ: Emotion, cognition, and behavior. Science 298:1191–1194, 2002

Ellsworth DL, Manolio TA: The emerging importance of genetics in epidemiologic research, III: bioinformatics and statistical genetic methods. Ann Epidemiol 9:207–224, 1999

Freedman RR, Ianni P, Ettedgui E, et al: Psychophysiological factors in panic disorder. Psychopathy 17(suppl):66–73, 1984

Galbaud du Fort G, Bland RC, Newman SC, et al: Spouse similarity for lifetime psychiatric history in the general population. Psychol Med 28:789–802, 1998

Gordis L: Epidemiology, 2nd Edition. Philadelphia, PA, WB Saunders, 2000

Gottesman I, Shields J: Schizophrenia and Genetics: A Twin Study Vantage Point. New York, Academic Press, 1972

Guttmacher AE, Collins FS: Genomic medicine: a primer. N Engl J Med 347:1512–1520, 2002

Hirschhorn JN, Lohmueller K, Byrne E, et al: A comprehensive review of genetic association studies. Genet Med 4:45–61, 2002

Hyman SE: The genetics of mental illness: implications for practice. Bull World Health Organ 78:455–463, 2000

Ishibe N, Kelsey KT: Genetic susceptibility to environmental and occupational cancers. Cancer Causes Control 8:504–513, 1997

Kendell RE: Clinical validity. Psychol Med 19:45–55, 1989

Kessler RC, Üstün TB: The World Health Organization World Mental Health 2000 Initiative. Hospital Management International 1:195–196, 2000

Kessler RC, McGonagle KA, Zhao S, et al: Lifetime and 12-month prevalence of DSM-III-R psychiatric disorders in the United States: results from the National Comorbidity Survey. Arch Gen Psychiatry 51:8–19, 1994

Khoury MJ, Dorman JS: The human genome epidemiology network. Am J Epidemiol 148:1–3, 1998

Khoury MJ, Yang Q: The future of genetic studies of complex human disease: an epidemiologic perspective. Epidemiology 9:350–354, 1998

Khoury MJ, McCabe LL, McCabe ER: Population screening in the age of genomic medicine. N Engl J Med 348:50–58, 2003

Levinson DF, Mowry BJ, Even K, et al: Genome scan of schizophrenia: results of genotyping of positive regions. Mol Psychiatry 4:S37, 1999

Maier W, Merikangas KR: Co-occurrence and co-transmission of affective disorders and alcoholism in families. Br J Psychiatry 168(suppl):93–100, 1996

Maier W, Lichtermann D, Minges J, et al: The relationship between bipolar disorder and alcoholism: a controlled family study. Psychol Med 25:787–796, 1995

McKhann GM: Neurology: then, now, and in the future. Arch Neurol 59:1369–1373, 2002

Merikangas KR: Assortative mating for psychiatric disorders and psychological traits. Arch Gen Psychiatry 39:1173–1180, 1982

Merikangas KR, Gelernter CS: Comorbidity for alcoholism and depression. Psychiatr Clin North Am 13:613–632, 1990

Merikangas KR, Swendsen J: Genetic epidemiology of psychiatric disorders. Epidemiol Rev 19:144–155, 1997

Merikangas KR, Rounsaville BJ, Prusoff BA: Familial factors in vulnerability to substance abuse, in Vulnerability to Drug Abuse. Edited by Glantz M, Pickens R. Washington, DC, American Psychological Association, 1992, pp 75–98, 1992

Merikangas KR, Angst J, Eaton W, et al: Comorbidity and boundaries of affective disorders with anxiety disorders and substance misuse: results of an international task force. Br J Psychiatry 168:58–67, 1996

Merikangas KR, Stevens DE, Fenton B, et al: Comorbidity and familial aggregation of alcoholism and anxiety disorders. Psychol Med 28:773–788, 1998

Merikangas KR, Chakravarti A, Moldin SO, et al: Future of genetics of mood disorders research: workgroup on genetics for NIMH strategic plan for mood disorders. Biol Psychiatry 52:457–477, 2002

Newman B, Millikan RC, King M: Genetic epidemiology of breast and ovarian cancers. Epidemiol Rev 19:69–79, 1997

Peltonen L, McKusick VA: Genomics and medicine: dissecting human disease in the postgenomic era. Science 291:1224–1229, 2001

Regier DA, Burke JD, Burke KC: Comorbidity of affective and anxiety disorders in the NIMH Epidemiologic Catchment Area (ECA) program, in Comorbidity of Mood and Anxiety Disorders. Edited by Maser JD, Cloninger CR. Washington, DC, American Psychiatric Press, 1990, pp 113–122

Risch N: Linkage strategies for genetically complex traits, I: multilocus models. Am J Hum Genet 46:222–228, 1990

Risch NJ: Searching for genetic determinants in the new millennium. Nature 405:847–856, 2000

Risch N, Merikangas KR: The future of genetic studies of complex human diseases. Science 273:1516–1517, 1996

St. George-Hyslop PH, McLaurin J, Fraser PE: Neuropathological, biochemical and genetic alterations in AD. Drug News Perspect 13:281–288, 2000

Thomas DC: Genetic epidemiology with a capital "E." Genet Epidemiol 19:289–300, 2000

Whittemore A: The Eighth AACR American Cancer Society Award lecture on cancer epidemiology and prevention. Genetically tailored preventive strategies: an effective plan for the twenty-first century? American Association for Cancer Research. Cancer Epidemiol Biomarkers Prev 8:649–658, 1999

Yang Q, Khoury MJ, Coughlin SC, et al: On the use of population-based registries in the clinical validation of genetic tests for disease susceptibility. Genet Med 2:186–192, 2000

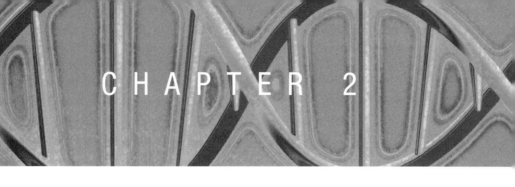

CHAPTER 2

New Genes for Human Behavior in Historical Perspective

Elliot S. Gershon, M.D.

The years 2002–2003 were a watershed for gene discovery in psychiatric disorders. After many years of false starts and unfulfilled promises, association of a series of genes with bipolar disorder and schizophrenia was reported, with each finding present in multiple data sets (Table 2–1). Moreover, the speculation based on linkage evidence that the same genes are involved in susceptibility to both disorders (Berrettini 2000; Gershon 2000; Wildenauer et al. 1999) was supported for the G72/G30 complex.

The findings on chromosomes 6, 8, and 13 underscore the validity of positional approaches (through linkage studies) to susceptibility gene identification. In a meta-analysis of all published genomewide linkage scans of bipolar disorder and schizophrenia, each region, with the exception of 6p, was found to have statistically significant linkage (Badner

Parts of this chapter are adapted from Gershon ES: "The Challenges of Genetic Tests for Human Behavior." *Israel Journal of Psychiatry and Related Sciences* 39:206–216, 2003. Used with permission.

TABLE 2–1.   Recent gene associations in psychiatric disorders

Gene	Location	Illness	Study
Dysbindin	6p	Schizophrenia	Straub et al. 2002
Neuregulin-1	8p	Schizophrenia	Stefansson et al. 2002, 2003
BDNF	11p	Bipolar disorder	Sklar et al. 2002
G72/G30	13q	Bipolar disorder, schizophrenia	Chumakov et al. 2002; Hattori et al. 2003

Note. BDNF=brain-derived neurotrophic factor.

and Gershon 2002a). The finding of a chromosomal linkage in a systematic meta-analysis, followed by significant association in several linked regions, underscores the validity of current positional approaches to complex disease inheritance, although there are still scholarly disputes among meta-analysts over which studies to include in their analyses. Linkage to schizophrenia on 6p was supported in several linkage studies that were not part of genomewide scans, so the association of schizophrenia with dysbindin also supports the positional approach.

Another region with significant linkage on meta-analysis in both bipolar disorder and schizophrenia is the long arm of chromosome 22. Here there have been numerous studies of the catechol-*O*-methyltransferase gene as a candidate in the right location, but a meta-analysis did not show support of association in either disorder (Lohmueller et al. 2003). Other candidates remain, including *GRK3* and *PRODh2*, but there is no definitive demonstration of the correct susceptibility variant in that region.

With several successes of consistency among linkage studies followed by consistent associations, and with some humility based on the fact that some of these new associations have been replicated only once, one must ask what went wrong previously. In retrospect, the failure to reproduce linkage of chromosomal markers to psychiatric disorders in the late 1980s can be attributed to inadequate genetic maps and inappropriate statistical analyses. For the field, the most devastating experience was the report of linkage of bipolar disorder to markers at the tip of the short arm of chromosome 11 in an extended Amish pedigree; in this study the statistical analysis was of a single major locus with variable penetrance (Egeland et al. 1987). This linkage was not replicated in follow-up of the original pedigree, after two individuals who, based on the linkage evidence, would not be at elevated risk became ill (Gershon and Goldin 1994; Kelsoe et al. 1989). No replications of this linkage have since been reported in other studies. The recent findings, on the other hand, have underlying linkages and subsequent associations each supported in multiple data sets, with analyses appropriate for complex inheritance common disease, using significantly enhanced genetic maps and genomic bioinformatics.

The association of brain-derived neurotrophic factor (BDNF) with bipolar disorder is based on a neurobiological candidate gene approach rather than a positional approach. These two approaches to disease gene identification in common disorders are both currently valid, although each has its partisans who occasionally disparage the other approach (Botstein and Risch 2003).

The astute reader may note that the BDNF gene is on the short arm of chromosome 11, as were the markers linked to bipolar disorder in the Amish pedigree. Yet the findings appear to be too far apart to be identical: the peak markers in the Amish pedigree are located about 25 million base pairs proximal to the BDNF gene on that chromosome (UCSC Genome Browser, Nov. 2002 freeze).

The statistical methods by which the current associations of genes with illness have been demonstrated are appropriate to the study of susceptibility genes that constitute risk factors for illness (as opposed to single genes that, acting alone, can independently cause disease). These genes are considered to have a "weak effect," because there is only a modest increase in the relative risk ratio associated with having the associated genotype. Thus, finding an individual within a pedigree who has the associated disease but not the associated haplotype or linked genotype is not, by itself, a refutation of an association or linkage. (Of course, frequent enough identification of such individuals *would* invalidate the finding.) Numerous modes of genetic transmission are compatible with these findings, including oligogenic inheritance with a few or with many genes conferring susceptibility.

The scientist may regret this ambiguity, because a single individual's genotype has little predictive power for the development of illness and yields insufficient power to test genetic hypotheses. However, as multiple associations of genes are established with each of the common psychiatric disorders, predictability of illness in individuals would become much more effective. From a political and historical perspective, research that may make psychiatric illnesses (and other illnesses) predictable awakens fears that advances in genetic knowledge will translate into discrimination against individuals and related fears of recrudescence of the eugenics movement as it played out in the nineteenth and twentieth centuries, with its horrendous treatment of individuals and groups thought to have undesirable genes.

THE HISTORICAL CONTEXT

Sir Francis Galton (1822–1911) is historically considered the founder of behavioral genetics as a scientific discipline, but he is also the founder of eugenics, a political and social movement that embodied the racial prejudices of his times and gave them a cloak of scientific respectability (Freeman 1983; Vogel and Motulsky 1986). *Eugenics* (usually translated as race improvement or racial hygiene) is a term introduced by Galton in 1883 and launched by him as a formal political movement in 1901. Its scientific basis is pre-Mendelian genetics, when inherited characteristics were not thought to sort independently. Rather, it was a nineteenth-century animal breeder's view of heredity—that an individual has more or less of the ideal characteristics of its breed (or its human race). Darwin's concepts of evolution were incorporated into this system of thought—human races were shaped by natural selection to be superior or inferior. Inferior races are primitive, apelike, and childlike as compared with superior races. Eugenics was seen as improvement of the superior race (not coincidentally, the race to which Galton belonged). Positive eugenics was encouragement of superior individuals of the superior race to mate together and breed. Negative eugenics was elimination of undesirable traits and inherited diseases, especially the feeble-minded and insane, from the superior race by preventing reproduction.

As an example of this perspective, the following passage appeared in a then-reputable human genetics textbook published in New York in 1931, in a translation from the German edition of 1927:

> In any case, there are close relationships between race and crime.... [The] "born criminal" belongs to a very special and primitive racial stock. Criminals very often exhibit characters which remind us of Neanderthal man or of other primitive races, having prominent and massive jaws, receding foreheads, etc. When a race is for the most part exterminated, or driven out, by another, there is nevertheless almost invariably some mingling of the bloods. (Baur et al. 1931, p. 681)

To the contemporary reader, scientific racism is an oxymoron, and the ideas advanced in the quoted text are reprehensible. They were controversial in their own day as well, but as a conflict of "nature versus nurture" (as Galton put it), in which a radical (and misinformed) view of the role of genetics in observed human variation was countered by a mirror-image environmentalist view (Table 2–2). The ideological conflicts of the Second World War were largely over these issues, rather than democracy versus totalitarianism as taught in the postwar history books.

TABLE 2–2.   Twentieth-century scientific and political extremism based on the nature versus nurture controversy

Philosophy	Genetic determinism	Sociocultural determinism
Political movement	Nazism	Communism (in Soviet Union)
Approved science	Eugenics (Galton), racial hygiene	Lamarckism, Marxist environmentalism (Lysenko)
Forbidden science	"Jewish" physics, "Jewish" psychiatry, any nonracist approaches in other disciplines	Genetics
Mass murder as implementation of science and philosophy	Murder of mentally ill Germans Genocide of Jews and Gypsies on racial grounds	Deliberate famine produced in Ukraine and elsewhere Murderous forced labor camps (gulags)

The political policies generated by adherents of the different ideologies can be seen as quite comparably extreme consequences of their opposite assumptions.

Although neither of these extreme outlooks has significant support today, an historical shadow has been cast over all current considerations of genetic differences among individuals, especially behavioral differences. As Steven Pinker (2002) noted,

> When it comes to explaining human thought and behavior, the possibility that heredity plays any role at all still has the power to shock. To acknowledge [heredity in] human nature, many think, is to endorse racism, sexism, war, greed, genocide, nihilism, reactionary politics, and neglect of children and the disadvantaged. (p. vii)

For contemporary citizens, including scientists and social policymakers, the historical reality of ideological racism makes it difficult to achieve a critical appreciation of scientific evidence on genetic variation. There is considerable reluctance to consider evidence from genetic studies of human behavior, with the partial exceptions of mental illnesses, retardation, and dementia. Genetic findings on "normal" human phenomena that are not part of a recognized illness, such as intelligence or sexual orientation, are usually controversial. Behaviors at the margin of normality, such as substance abuse or those associated with antisocial per-

sonality, are subject to considerable public debate over whether any genetic component could legitimately exist.

Given the twentieth century's history of great mischief perpetrated
in the name of genetic differences, it is understandable when reports
that such differences exist are questioned or denied. Nonetheless, if scientific evidence continues to progress toward identification of widely
distributed inherited components of mental illnesses and undesired behaviors, hard questions will be raised on whether it is justified to categorize individuals by these genes. The obvious answer is no, unless there
are expected beneficial effects for the individual being tested, but there
is room for controversy within this answer. From the viewpoint of science policy, however, the question of whether to support research on
such differences is not a simple one, because there are potential benefits
of treatment based on genetic knowledge and because of the potential
of such research to illuminate more general questions, such as the mind–
body problem.

POTENTIAL FOR EFFECTIVE GENETIC DISCRIMINATION BASED ON COMMON DISEASE SUSCEPTIBILITY ALLELES

Numerous single-gene diseases have clearly elucidated causes; the first
such psychiatric disease was phenylketonuria, where the phenolic odor
of the urine of two retarded brothers led to the discovery, in 1934, of excess
metabolites of phenylalanine in their urine (Folling 1934). Phenylketonuria is a simple inheritance recessive disease, and it is generally screened
for in neonates and treated fairly effectively by diet during infancy and
childhood. However, if we consider mental retardation as the disease,
then phenylketonuria is only one of the subtypes included, and there
are many different inheritance patterns of the different subtypes. A substantial proportion of the subtypes of mental retardation fit this model:
"true genetic heterogeneity" of independent single-gene disorders with
a common clinical presentation. As a contrast, and for simplicity, I lump
together as "oligogenic inheritance" all the inheritance patterns in which
two or more separate genes are needed to generate a substantial probability of illness in an individual. This type of inheritance is generally
agreed to apply in schizophrenia (Risch 1990) and bipolar illness.

There are known examples of each type of inheritance in common
disease. True genetic heterogeneity is found in Alzheimer's disease, in
which there are rare single-gene variants located on chromosomes 21,
14, and 1, and in breast carcinoma, with single-gene forms on chromo-

somes 17 and 13. A much more frequent susceptibility allele for Alzheimer's disease than the single-gene forms is *APOE4* (allele 4 of the gene for apolipoprotein E), which is part of the oligogenic inheritance of the common form of the illness and was the first risk factor reported for a common neuropsychiatric disease (Strittmatter et al. 1993). Recently, genes that are part of oligenic susceptibility for non–insulin-dependent diabetes mellitus (NIDDM) and inflammatory bowel disease (IBD) have been reported, as discussed below.

Let us consider stigmatization in view of these two modes of inheritance and ask whether stigmatization of gene carriers would be effective in achieving its goal (of distancing the stigmatizer from a disease). For example, a potential employer or a potential spouse might wish to discriminate on that basis. This question is not raised to justify stigma but to consider if there are incentives for stigmatization. For oligogenically inherited disease, most of the phenotypic expression of any single susceptibility allele will not be illness. If stigma were applied rationally, it would not often be applied to persons with one susceptibility allele of one gene. One may ask, what if all susceptibility alleles of all involved genes could be identified in an individual? Identical twins of patients with oligogenic inheritance common disease do not all show illness, which may be interpreted to mean that even a complete set of susceptibility alleles is not sufficient to produce disease (although an alternative explanation would be that some illness is not genetic). Nonetheless, if one could genotype for all the susceptibility genes for an illness like schizophrenia, this procedure would be expected to identify persons with approximately the same risk for schizophrenia as an identical twin (just under 50%). It would be a valid, if inefficient, predictor.

Stigma on the basis of family history in an oligogenic inheritance disease would *not* be notably effective. The relative risk (ratio of risk to a sibling to the population risk) is typically 1,000 or more for a rare single-gene disease but much smaller (typically 3–5) for complex inheritance common disease. A family history of illness does give a modest basis for avoiding the specific disease (in a prospective employee or in having children with a particular spouse), but the overall protective effect to the stigmatizer is evanescent. There exist such a large number of common diseases that eventually, nearly every person will have one or more. A choice of employee or spouse based on family history might weakly avoid a risk of one disease but may not appreciably reduce the risk that some common disease or diseases will eventually strike the alternative person chosen, or his or her children.

This point is particularly pertinent to members of some communities with arranged marriages, in which family history of psychiatric illness is a major disqualification for a potential match. This practice reflects an extreme and irrational stigma associated with these disorders. The modest gains from avoiding a potential spouse with a family history of mental illness, in terms of the disease risk avoided, must be weighed against the loss of the personal qualities that made the potential spouse considered in the first place and against the overall likelihood of any common disease not being appreciably changed.

COMMON DISEASE: CURRENT FINDINGS

From the recent successes in discovering susceptibility associations based on linkage and on neurobiological candidate genes, it is reasonable to expect that all the common susceptibility alleles for these psychiatric disorders will be discovered in the foreseeable future and that it will be possible to test individuals for susceptibility. To put the psychiatric data in context with other common disease genetic findings, consider the report of a causal connection between *Calpain-10* mutations and increased susceptibility to NIDDM (Horikawa et al. 2000). This finding, which included important statistical methodological advances (Cox et al. 1999), demonstrated the plausibility of applying currently feasible experimental, statistical, and computational tools to the successful identification of complex disease genes, starting with a linkage result. This discovery was made despite the usual complications of complex disease genetics—apparently inconsistent linkage results, study of an outbred population, and no obvious candidate genes in the linkage region. The keys to the discovery were innovative and meticulous analysis of disequilibrium in a sample of families with a positive linkage result and thorough molecular scrutiny of the disequilibrium region.

The pedigree studied by Horikawa et al. (2000) is the only known sample with significant linkage evidence for NIDDM in this region of chromosome 2 (Hanis et al. 1996). It is a sample from an outbred Mexican-American population, one of four samples studied in that report. There exist two other major linkage reports: a report from a French sample that does not reach significance but provides modest nominal support for linkage (*P* values roughly 0.01–0.07), and a large multinational study that is not at all positive (Ghosh et al. 1998; Hani et al. 1997). Meta-analysis of all samples from all published linkage reports using a chromosomal-region adaptation of Fisher's meta-analysis test (Badner and Gershon 2002b) gives a *P* value for the linkage of 5.6×10^{-5}, which in retrospect supports the approach taken by the NIDDM researchers.

In IBD, a linkage finding on chromosome 16 followed by disequilibrium studies of the region led to discovery of susceptibility mutations in the *NOD2* gene (Hugot et al. 2001; Ogura et al. 2001). Prior to this finding, linkage to chromosome 16 was reported in several studies with varying levels of significance and at varying markers (Annese et al. 1999; Brant et al. 1998; Cavanaugh et al. 1998; Hampe et al. 1999; Hugot et al. 1996; Mirza et al. 1998; Ohmen et al. 1996; Parkes et al. 1996). However, not all studies demonstrated linkage, despite similar sample sizes in the studies that did report linkage (Duerr et al. 2000; Rioux et al. 1998; Vermeire et al. 2000).

The status of linkage data in these diseases prior to gene discovery was one of apparent inconsistency between studies, although a consistent conclusion could be reached through meta-analysis. The situation of linkage data in bipolar disorder and schizophrenia a few years ago is strikingly reminiscent of the earlier status of linkage in IBD and NIDDM. In retrospect, this situation was not sufficient reason to discourage attempts, based on the positive linkage samples, to discover susceptibility genes.

Prediction of risk will be practical only when multiple genes have been identified, as discussed earlier, because each gene confers little change in risk. The phenotypic expressions of susceptibility genes for psychiatric disorders may well include the whole spectrum of behaviors that aggregate in families of patients (i.e., are more frequent in families of patients than in control subjects). Immediate relatives of bipolar patients have increased frequency of bipolar disorder, recurrent major depression, schizoaffective disorder, and suicide without prior diagnosis. Yet the observed spectrum in patients and relatives also includes increased artistic achievement, particularly in literature and music; historical leaders; religious leaders; media magnates; and other socially outstanding individuals. These achievements must be borne in mind in considering how to respond to genetic vulnerability to illness—that is, increased power of prediction of risk for illness will come with increased complexity of the predictions themselves.

Subsequent goals of research, following discovery of susceptibility genes, would be therapeutic advances. These advances would follow from increased understanding of the pathophysiology of illness and of treatment side effects, which would follow from identification of the genes involved (a classic progression in reverse genetics). Gene therapy might eventually be one of the therapeutic modalities developed, depending on the timing of the gene's pathophysiological role.

THE CHALLENGES

The historical examples of racism based on archaic and mistaken genetic concepts of character, intelligence, and inherited mental disorders generate legitimate concern that advances in risk prediction could lead to stigmatization of individuals based on their genotypes and stigmatization of whole communities based on allele frequencies. There is also a mirror-image hazard associated with stigmatization, namely anti-stigmatization, or ennoblement, of persons or communities based on their allele frequencies. The history of eugenics and racism in the nineteenth and twentieth centuries gives ample evidence that this sort of narcissistic enhancement goes hand-in-hand with a sense of unbridled entitlement and a capacity for great evil.

Nonetheless, one cannot avoid the evil by suppressing the science, because rationalizations for evil may be found in the absence of good scientific knowledge, as they have been in the past. A constructive approach of understanding and anticipating the dangers may be what is needed to prevent their materializing. From the societal viewpoint, in addition to an acute historical awareness of the potential for mischief based on genetics, consideration of specific areas in which prejudicial discrimination may occur is required. Such areas include decisions on health care, insurance, and employment. One can envision legislative remedies to such discrimination, and in the United States there have been several legislative initiatives to achieve such remedies, so far without significant success. But I am optimistic successful initiatives will come to pass. Decisions on marriage and childbearing, however, may become greatly influenced by genetic considerations in an era when susceptibility to multiple diseases can be identified. These decisions would not be regulated by legislation, nor ought they to be, in view of the history of the eugenics movement.

The question of abortion of pregnancies in which the fetus is at increased risk of a medical disorder or stigmatized trait in adult life has been raised repeatedly in public discussions, as in the off Broadway play *The Twilight of the Golds,* in which a couple learns that the woman is carrying a child who will be homosexual. The caveats noted earlier on the precision of risk prediction and the losses to humanity of people who have normal or extraordinary human potential during much of their lives must inform the public debate and the private deliberations of prospective parents. There is no ethical consensus now, in Western societies, on how to proceed when genotypic predictions of complex traits become possible.

A Contemporary Response to Genetic Risks by
Ultra-Orthodox Jews

Marriage negotiations, if informed by valid genetic risk information, could generate the same discrimination and stigmatization as could less intimate decisions, such as health care access. Persons at risk for illness might become unmarriageable. On the other hand, there may be an un-avoidable incentive to avoid having a deadly illness in one's spouse or children. The ethics of marriage choice, and the culture necessary to avoid human tragedies as a result of genetic testing, are currently evolving. I am aware of one culture that has successfully addressed some of these issues, the ultra-Orthodox Ashkenazi Jewish community, and their solu-tion may provide some insight toward devising more general solutions.

In this community, marriages are arranged, with some limited public meetings prior to confirming the match. Family history is a major factor in premarital negotiations, both for positive qualities and for disease. Diseases affecting the nervous system are particularly stigmatized in these negotiations. The pertinent religious precepts are that everyone should marry (if they are competent to do so) and that abortion is a form of mayhem and is to be avoided, except for very unusual circumstances. The prevailing rabbinic opinion is that abortion of a Tay-Sachs fetus is not justifiable (Bleich 1977), yet the prevalence of carriers for this reces-sive disease is much higher among Ashkenazi Jews than in most other populations.

In the context of these facts, a movement has arisen within this com-munity to reduce the frequency of Tay-Sachs births as well as that of some other recessive diseases. The ingenuity of the solution is that it achieves its goals, follows community norms, *and* avoids stigma to the carriers. A voluntary community agency, Dor Yesharim, collects blood specimens from adolescents within the community. The adolescents and their family receive an identification code at the time the specimens are collected, but no test results. The specimens and data are kept com-pletely outside the health care system and do not constitute a medical record. When a marriage is contemplated, each family gives its code num-ber to the agency, and one of two possible responses are given: either "Nothing is known to us that would advise against the match," or "There is a reason to be concerned about this match." In the event of the latter comment, if the contemplated match is dropped, neither party is bur-dened by having a test result that he or she is a carrier for a specific dis-ease. Under the norms of the community, they are therefore not obliged to disclose a condition to another prospective spouse. Also, the couple has generally not yet formed deep attachments to each other, so the grief upon ending the marriage possibility is minimal.

There are many genetic problems not solved by this approach, such as that of the person who herself has a dominant disease gene (such as for breast cancer) or has a pre-mutation so that her offspring is at high risk whomever she marries (such as fragile X mental retardation). Yet the principles of avoiding stigma, and of attempting to make it possible for a person with unfortunate test results to marry and have children, are surely of general applicability.

Screening Issues

Although there is a greater yield of true positives from screening relatives of persons with known cases of a disease than from screening the population, there is considerably less psychological trauma and fewer soured family relationships to be expected from the latter choice. Also, for diseases for which the family history is a very imperfect guide to detecting persons at risk, only exhaustive screening of the population will serve to greatly reduce illness.

Not all diseases whose genes are detectable should be the subject of screening, as noted earlier. A considered decision has to be made—one that takes into account the value of screening (in terms of illnesses prevented), its costs (psychological and social as well as economic), the actions that may be taken as a result of positive results, the desirability of those actions, and the likelihood and costs of false-positive and false-negative test results. A case in point is the *APOE* ε4 allele that is predictive of increased risk for Alzheimer's disease. In Caucasians, the risk in late-onset familial Alzheimer's disease is up to 90% with the allele and 20% without it, and the age at onset is 16 years earlier (Corder et al. 1993). More recent estimates of the penetrance, however, are much lower (Molero et al. 2001). The disease is greatly feared. The medical consensus is not to test, because the distress of a positive result appears greater than the benefit. Nonetheless, when a person strongly desires testing and can give informed consent for it, his or her request should not be denied.

CONCLUSION

There are a host of behavioral traits with evidence for significant heritability, including intelligence (as measured by IQ), reading disability, and personality dimensions (McGuffin et al. 2001). On the borders between psychopathology and undesirable behavior, there is evidence for heritability of criminal behavior (Hutchings and Mednick 1975; Mednick et al. 1984) and alcoholism (Cloninger et al. 1978). The same possibilities for use and misuse of genotype data would apply to these traits, once genes are identified, as to psychiatric disorder. The history of the eugenics movement offers considerable caution to us today. It is difficult to conceive of any positive value of genotyping for these traits at their multiple susceptibility loci, if the only purpose is to categorize individuals. However, one can reasonably anticipate that identification of genotypes could lead to remedial and preventive education and treatment modalities and that these developments could proceed without stigmatization of individuals.

In general, there are reasons to be cautious about the development of clinical genetic tests as applications of the genotypic associations with human behavior that are on the scientific horizon. Even when diagnostic tests have clear benefit to the persons tested, or to persons yet to be born, the costs will need to be borne in mind. These include the burden of genotypic data as a new dimension of a person's sense of identity and self-worth, the potential for stigmatization of individuals and communities, and the increased medical costs of employing genetic technology for human benefits. The potential for misuse of genotype data on behavior traits as well as on psychiatric disorders cannot be dismissed, but it can be guarded against. My own outlook is that the potential benefits of new knowledge, including treatments, far outweigh the dangers of misapplication in a society determined to learn from and to avoid the extremism of the past.

REFERENCES

Annese V, Latiano A, Bovio P, et al: Genetic analysis in Italian families with inflammatory bowel disease supports linkage to the IBD1 locus: a GISC study. Eur J Hum Genet 7:567–573, 1999

Badner JA, Gershon ES: Meta-analysis of whole-genome linkage scans of bipolar disorder and schizophrenia. Mol Psychiatry 7:405–411, 2002a

Badner JA, Gershon ES: Regional meta-analysis of published data supports linkage of autism with markers on chromosome 7. Mol Psychiatry 7:56–66, 2002b

Baur B, Fischer E, Lenz F: Human Heredity. New York, MacMillan, 1931

Berrettini WH: Susceptibility loci for bipolar disorder: overlap with inherited vulnerability to schizophrenia. Biol Psychiatry 47:245–251, 2000

Bleich JD: Contemporary Halakhic Problems. New York, Yeshiva University Press/ Ktav Publishing, 1977

Botstein D, Risch N: Discovering genotypes underlying human phenotypes: past successes for mendelian disease, future approaches for complex disease. Nat Genet 33(suppl):228–237, 2003

Brant SR, Fu Y, Fields CT, et al: American families with Crohn's disease have strong evidence for linkage to chromosome 16 but not chromosome 12. Gastroenterology 115:1056–1061, 1998

Cavanaugh JA, Callen DF, Wilson SR, et al: Analysis of Australian Crohn's disease pedigrees refines the localization for susceptibility to inflammatory bowel disease on chromosome 16. Ann Hum Genet 62:291–298, 1998

Chumakov I, Blumenfeld M, Guerassimenko O, et al: Genetic and physiological data implicating the new human gene G72 and the gene for D-amino acid oxidase in schizophrenia. Proc Natl Acad Sci U S A 99:13675–13680, 2002

Cloninger CR, Christiansen KO, Reich T, et al: Implications of sex differences in the prevalences of antisocial personality, alcoholism, and criminality for familial transmission. Arch Gen Psychiatry 35:941–951, 1978

Corder EH, Saunders AM, Strittmatter WJ, et al: Gene dose of apolipoprotein E type 4 allele and the risk of Alzheimer's disease in late onset families (see comments). Science 261:921–923, 1993

Cox NJ, Frigge M, Nicolae DL, et al: Loci on chromosomes 2 (NIDDM1) and 15 interact to increase susceptibility to diabetes in Mexican Americans. Nat Genet 21:213–215, 1999

Duerr RH, Barmada MM, Zhang L, et al: High-density genome scan in Crohn's disease shows confirmed linkage to chromosome 14q11–12. Am J Hum Genet 66:1857–1862, 2000

Egeland JA, Gerhard DS, Pauls DL, et al: Bipolar affective disorders linked to DNA markers on chromosome 11. Nature 325:783–787, 1987

Folling A: Ueber ausscheidung von phenylbrenztraubensaeure in den harn als stoffwechselanomalie in verbindung mit imbezillitaet. Ztschr Physiol Chem 227:169–176, 1934

Freeman D: Margaret Mead and Samoa: The Making and Unmaking of an Anthropological Myth. Cambridge, MA, Harvard University Press, 1983

Gershon ES: Bipolar illness and schizophrenia as oligogenic diseases: implications for the future. Biol Psychiatry 47:240–244, 2000

Gershon ES, Goldin LR: Replication of genetic linkage by follow-up of previously studied pedigrees. Am J Hum Genet 54:715–718, 1994

Ghosh S, Hauser ER, Magnuson VL, et al: A large sample of Finnish diabetic sib pairs reveals no evidence for a non-insulin-dependent diabetes mellitus susceptibility locus at 2qter. J Clin Invest 102:704–709, 1998

Hampe J, Schreiber S, Shaw SH, et al: A genomewide analysis provides evidence for novel linkages in inflammatory bowel disease in a large European cohort. Am J Hum Genet 64:808–816, 1999

Hani EH, Hager J, Philippi A, et al: Mapping NIDDM susceptibility loci in French families: studies with markers in the region of NIDDM1 on chromosome 2q. Diabetes 46:1225–1226, 1997

Hanis CL, Boerwinkle E, Chakraborty R, et al: A genome-wide search for human non-insulin-dependent (type 2) diabetes genes reveals a major susceptibility locus on chromosome 2 (see comments). Nat Genet 13:161–166, 1996

Hattori E, Liu C, Badner JA, et al: Polymorphisms at the G72/G30 gene locus on 13q33 are associated with bipolar disorder in two independent pedigree series. Am J Hum Genet 72:1131–1140, 2003

Horikawa Y, Oda N, Cox NJ, et al: Genetic variation in the gene encoding calpain-10 is associated with type 2 diabetes mellitus. Nat Genet 26:163–175, 2000

Hugot JP, Laurent-Puig P, Gower-Rousseau C, et al: Mapping of a susceptibility locus for Crohn's disease on chromosome 16. Nature 379:821–823, 1996

Hugot JP, Chammaillard M, Zouali H, et al: Association of NOD2 leucine-rich repeat variants with susceptibility to Crohn's disease. Nature 411:599–603, 2001

Hutchings B, Mednick SA: Registered criminality in the adoptive and biological parents of registered male criminal adoptees. Proc Annu Meet Am Psychopathol Assoc 63:105–116, 1975

Kelsoe JR, Ginns EI, Egeland JA, et al: Re-evaluation of the linkage relationship between chromosome 11p loci and the gene for bipolar affective disorder in the Old Order Amish. Nature 342:238–243, 1989

Lohmueller KE, Pearce CL, Pike M, et al: Meta-analysis of genetic association studies supports a contribution of common variants to susceptibility to common disease. Nat Genet 33:177–182, 2003

McGuffin P, Riley B, Plomin R: Genomics and behavior: toward behavioral genomics. Science 291:1232–1249, 2001

Mednick SA, Gabrielli WF Jr, Hutchings B: Genetic influences in criminal convictions: evidence from an adoption cohort. Science 224:891–894, 1984

Mirza MM, Lee J, Teare D, et al: Evidence of linkage of the inflammatory bowel disease susceptibility locus on chromosome 16 (IBD1) to ulcerative colitis. J Med Genet 35:218–221, 1998

Molero AE, Pino-Ramirez G, Maestre GE: Modulation by age and gender of risk for Alzheimer's disease and vascular dementia associated with the apolipoprotein E-var epsilon4 allele in Latin Americans: findings from the Maracaibo Aging Study. Neurosci Lett 307:5–8, 2001

Ogura Y, Bonen DK, Inohara N, et al: A frameshift mutation in NOD2 associated with susceptibility to Crohn's disease. Nature 411:603–606, 2001

Ohmen JD, Yang HY, Yamamoto KK, et al: Susceptibility locus for inflammatory bowel disease on chromosome 16 has a role in Crohn's disease, but not in ulcerative colitis. Hum Mol Genet 5:1679–1683, 1996

Parkes M, Satsangi J, Lathrop GM, et al: Susceptibility loci in inflammatory bowel disease. Lancet 348:1588, 1996

Pinker S: The Blank Slate: The Modern Denial of Human Nature. New York, Penguin Putnam, 2002

Rioux JD, Daly MJ, Green T, et al: Absence of linkage between inflammatory bowel disease and selected loci on chromosomes 3, 7, 12, and 16. Gastroenterology 115:1062–1065, 1998

Risch N: Linkage strategies for genetically complex traits, I: multilocus models. Am J Hum Genet 46:222–228, 1990

Sklar P, Gabriel SB, McInnis MG, et al: Family-based association study of 76 candidate genes in bipolar disorder: BDNF is a potential risk locus. Mol Psychiatry 7:579–593, 2002

Stefansson H, Sigurdsson E, Steinthorsdottir V, et al: Neuregulin 1 and susceptibility to schizophrenia. Am J Hum Genet 71:877–892, 2002

Stefansson H, Sarginson J, Kong A, et al: Association of neuregulin 1 with schizophrenia confirmed in a Scottish population. Am J Hum Genet 72:83–87, 2003

Straub RE, Jiang Y, MacLean CJ, et al: Genetic variation in the 6p22.3 gene DTNBP1, the human ortholog of the mouse dysbindin gene, is associated with schizophrenia. Am J Hum Genet 71:337–348, 2002

Strittmatter WJ, Weber JL, Pericak-Vance MA, et al: Apolipoprotein E: high avidity binding to beta-amyloid and increased frequency of type 4 isoform in late-onset familial Alzheimer disease. Proc Natl Acad Sci U S A 90:1977–1981, 1993

Vermeire S, Peeters M, Vlietinck R, et al: Exclusion of linkage of Crohn's disease to previously reported regions on chromosomes 12, 7, and 3 in the Belgian population indicates genetic heterogeneity. Inflamm Bowel Dis 6:165–170, 2000

Vogel F, Motulsky AG: Human Genetics: Problems and Approaches. Berlin, Germany, Springer-Verlag, 1986

Wildenauer DB, Schwab SG, Maier W, et al: Do schizophrenia and affective disorder share susceptibility genes? Schizophr Res 39:107–111, 1999

CHAPTER 3

Redefining
Early-Onset Disorders
for Genetic Studies

Attention-Deficit/Hyperactivity Disorder
and Autism

Richard D. Todd, Ph.D., M.D.

John N. Constantino, M.D.

Rosalind J. Neuman, Ph.D.

The twenty-first century will see the reconceptualization of medicine and medical diagnoses to include molecular genetic components. For psychopathological disorders to be included in these advances, our nosology needs to become both biologically and genetically meaningful. Many of these issues were discussed at length in the American Psychopathological Association Series book *Defining Psychopathology in the Twenty-First Century: DSM-V and Beyond* (Helzer and Hudziak 2002). The goal of this chapter is to describe specific experimental approaches that can inform revisions of psychiatric nosology and demonstrate their application to two early-onset disorders, attention-deficit/hyperactivity disorder (ADHD) and autism.

At the heart of any nosology are the concepts of what is a *disease* and what is a *syndrome*. In most definitions of a *disease*, a specific pathological agent, such as a microbe, a toxin, or a genetic mutation, can be identified. With rare exception, the major psychiatric disorders have no well-established etiological agents. Hence, most of our diagnoses are syndromatic. In its most basic form the definition of a *syndrome* is a collection of signs and symptoms that occur together more frequently than expected by chance. Hence, psychiatric diagnosis at the present time should be based on epidemiological and statistical data. Despite these well-known concepts, few psychiatric syndromes meet these criteria due to a lack of attention to the prevalence and clustering of individual symptoms and signs in the general population. For rare serious disorders, which essentially always come to clinical attention, a lack of epidemiologically based data may have relatively limited impact on the definition of a syndrome. On the other hand, relying on clinically ascertained signs and symptoms for common and non-incapacitating disorders can give very misleading conceptualizations of key features of disorders. For example, the long-standing shortage of child and adolescent psychiatrists results in the preferential referral for evaluation and treatment of children who tend to have more serious or comorbid forms of a given disorder. This situation in part has given rise to the concept of autism being a very extreme categorical disorder and to the concept of combined subtype ADHD (i.e., ADHD with prominent inattentive and hyperactive impulsive symptoms) being the most common form of ADHD. As is described in the following summary of our epidemiologically based studies, both of these concepts are likely to be incorrect.

In the remainder of this chapter we describe results from population-based studies of ADHD and autism symptoms using the same general experimental approach. In each case, psychiatric assessments were completed for population-based samples of children and adolescents by collecting data on *all* symptoms suggested in DSM-IV-TR (American Psychiatric Association 2000) and related constructs. The collection of data on all symptoms in an epidemiological framework allows the unbiased application of factor analytic and clustering techniques to determine what constellations of symptoms occur more frequently in individuals than expected by chance. This approach also allows us to test, at least in a preliminary way, whether continuum models of risk or categorical diagnoses are more appropriate frameworks for our basic nosology. In both sets of analyses we have collected data from population-based samples of twins. Such data allows the testing of whether population-based syndromes represent appropriate phenotypes for studies aimed at discovering genetic variations that contribute to risk.

DESCRIPTION OF SAMPLES FOR ANALYSIS

Although some of the studies to be described included clinically ascertained samples to test certain hypotheses, the majority of our work is involved in the application of diagnostic interviews and questionnaires to population-based sample of twins. The three twin samples we have utilized to date are described in Table 3–1. The Missouri Adolescent Female Twin Study (MOAFTS; Andrew Heath, principal investigator) involved parent and adolescent interviews on approximately 2,400 twin pairs ages 11–17 years at the time of initial contact. The overall goal of this study is to determine antecedents of drug and alcohol abuse in women. The Missouri Twin Study (MOTWINS; Richard Todd, principal investigator) is a two-stage twin study designed to determine what components of ADHD are heritable. In this study, 5,000 families of children ages 7–18 years were screened for ADHD symptoms. Those meeting a screening criterion were then invited for personal interviews. In addition to evaluating for DSM-IV (American Psychiatric Association 1994) symptoms, the investigators obtained measures of IQ, academic performance, and reciprocal social behavior for this sample. Finally, many of the initial findings from the MOTWINS were replicated in the Australian Twin ADHD Project (ATAP; David Hay and Florence Levy, principal investigators). This voluntary birth record registry is largely representative of youth in Australia. In contrast to the telephone or personal interviews of the Missouri studies, all diagnostic assessments were done via mailed questionnaire.

ANALYTIC FRAMEWORK FOR ALL STUDIES

To test for clustering of symptoms in these general population samples as well as to test whether categorical or dimensional models best described symptom clusters, we performed a similar series of analyses for ADHD and autism symptoms. In each case we applied factor-analytic and latent-class analysis of symptom reports followed by comparisons of monozygotic and dizygotic twins to test for the familiality and heritability of the derived symptom clusters. In ongoing studies we are using the derived symptom clusters to look at different covariants across groups such as psychiatric comorbidity, alcohol and drug use, and educational performance.

Factor-analytic analysis is a widely used statistical procedure in which the interrelationships among a set of observed variables are postulated to be due to a small number of underlying continuous unobserved (latent)

TABLE 3–1. Description of twin samples

	MOAFTS	MOTWINS	ATAP
Sampling frame	All live twin births	Two stage, all live twin births	Voluntary birth registry
Participation rates	92% with one informant	Stage 1=94%; Stage 2=63%	78% of original sample at ages 7–17 years
Diagnostic assessments	C-SSAGA, DICA-R based	MAGIC, CBCL, WISC-III, WRAT-R, SRS	DSM-IV parent questionnaire

Note. ATAP=Australian Twin ADHD Project; C-SSAGA=Semi-Structured Assessment for the Genetics of Alcoholism, Child Version; CBCL=Child Behavior Checklist; DICA-R= Diagnostic Interview for Children and Adolescents—Revised; MAGIC=Missouri Assessment of Genetics Interview for Children; MOAFTS=Missouri Adolescent Female Twin Study; MOTWINS=Missouri Twin Study; SRS=Social Reciprocity Scale; WISC-III= Wechsler Intelligence Scale for Children–III; WRAT-R=Wide Range Achievement Test—Revised.

variables known as *factors*. In contrast, latent-class analysis uses categorical data to identify an underlying latent variable with a finite number of mutually exclusive classes that would explain the observed association. Furthermore, this underlying latent variable may be characterized as defining either a set of distinct categories (or typologies) or a continuum of categories within the dataset. For a given latent-class model, the conditional probabilities describing the distribution of the endorsement for each observed variable on the symptom can be depicted graphically. As seen in the top panel of Figure 3–1, the symptom endorsement profiles (in this case, symptoms A through I in the figure) seem to identify two distinct patterns of response or two distinct subtypes. In contrast, if the true model is an underlying continuum, then if more than one class is derived, the symptom endorsement profiles for the different classes will appear parallel—that is, they will all have the same shape but differ only by the average level of symptom endorsement probability for each class (i.e., the classes will differ only in the severity of given symptom endorsements [bottom of figure]). Because there are no formal statistical tests to determine whether continuum or categorical models best fit data, such graphical guidelines can be useful in weighing the relative merits of each diagnostic structure.

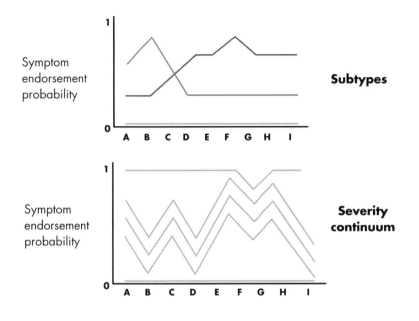

Symptom endorsement probability   **Subtypes**

Symptom endorsement probability   **Severity continuum**

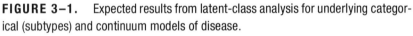

FIGURE 3–1.   Expected results from latent-class analysis for underlying categorical (subtypes) and continuum models of disease.

A through I represent individual symptoms or signs.

The final latent-class model can be used to test whether the data are compatible with a genetic contribution to the symptom complex. Under the hypothesis of a genetic component, monozygotic twins should be assigned to the same latent class more often than dizygotic twins, particularly in the case of a categorical structure to the data (Figure 3–1, top). However, if a continuum model fits the data, the sibling recurrence concordance in latent-class assignment may be "spread" across adjacent latent classes (Figure 3–1, bottom).

POPULATION-BASED ANALYSIS OF ADHD SYMPTOMS

Our first attempt at analyzing ADHD data was with the MOAFTS (Hudziak et al. 1998; Neuman et al. 1999; Todd 2001). In our most complete presentation, we analyzed the 18 DSM-IV ADHD symptoms reported by parents for 4,036 female twins age 13–23 years. Factor analysis was most compatible with there being three dimensions of ADHD symptoms (attention problems, hyperactivity/impulsivity problems, and combined problems factors) (Hudziak et al. 1998). This result is largely in keeping with findings from previous studies of the factor structure of ADHD. Latent-class analysis was most compatible with the existence of eight ADHD subtypes (Figure 3–2). Two classes had relatively high endorsement of hyperactive/impulsive symptoms versus inattentive symptoms. Two classes had high endorsement of inattentive symptoms and very low endorsement of hyperactive/impulsive symptoms. Two other classes showed high endorsement of all symptoms, and one class showed an idiosyncratic pattern of high endorsement of the "talks excessively" symptom as well as the impulsivity symptoms. The most common class showed low endorsement of all symptoms. There was moderate overlap between the three most severe latent classes and the DSM-IV-defined ADHD subtypes. DSM-IV-defined primarily inattentive and combined subtypes of ADHD co-clustered within families in the MOAFTS sample, suggesting a lack of genetic specificity for these subtypes (Todd et al. 2001). In contrast, the primarily hyperactive/impulsive DSM-IV subtype did not cluster with the other two. All eight latent-class-defined ADHD subtypes showed no evidence of co-clustering within families. All the subtypes showed very high monozygotic/dizygotic concordance rates, suggesting that latent-class-defined ADHD is both highly heritable and likely to be categorical in nature. In an extension of these studies, the basic-eight latent-class solution was confirmed in the ATAP. Of importance, in the ATAP we could also demonstrate that the same class structure was present for boys and for girls and non-twin siblings (Rasmussen et al. 2002). In this study we also demonstrated high heritability of the individual latent-class subtypes and lack of co-clustering of latent-class subtypes (Rasmussen et al. 2004). As shown in Table 3–2 for both the MOAFTS and ATAP families, the only significant odds ratios for monozygotic/dizygotic concordance for the ADHD latent classes were for same class membership.

The most parsimonious explanation for these data is that there are discrete categories of ADHD symptom clusters in the general population for both children and adolescents and for both boys and girls. Three of these classes superficially resemble the subtypes defined in DSM-IV- and DSM-IV-TR. Interestingly, analyses of school performance in the MOTWINS sample demonstrate not only marked impairment in these severe symptom classes but also significant impairment in latent classes with less severe endorsement of inattentive problems. This finding, which could not be explained by the presence of learning disabilities or cognitive impairment, suggests, from the point of view of school education,

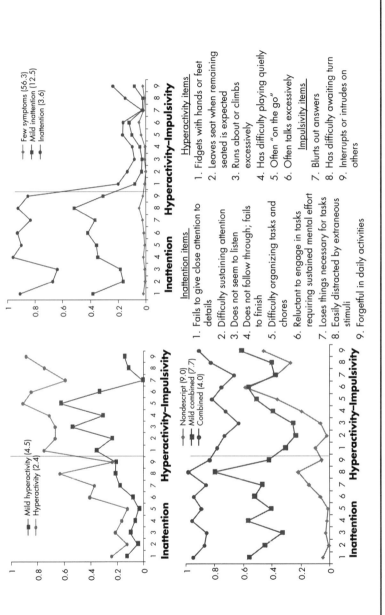

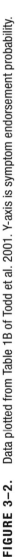

FIGURE 3–2. Data plotted from Table 1B of Todd et al. 2001. Y-axis is symptom endorsement probability.

TABLE 3–2. Same- and cross-class odds ratios for monozygotic/dizygotic concordance for attention-deficit/hyperactivity disorder latent classes (MOAFTS and ATAP)

Class	1 Few	2 Mild Inattentive	3 Inattentive Impulsive	4 Talkative Impulsive	5 Severe Inattentive	6 Severe Combined	7 Severe Hyperimpulsive	8 Unique
1 Few	1.4 / 17							
2 Mild inattentive		2.1 / 1.9						
3 Inattentive impulsive			3.2 / 1.6					
4 Talkative impulsive				3.0 / 4.1				
5 Severe inattentive					6.0 / 2.2			
6 Severe combined						3.2 / 3.0		
7 Severe hyperimpulsive							36.9 / 2.4	
8 Unique								5.7 / 2.1

Note. Only significant odds ratios above 1.0 are shown. All values are age, sex, and ethnicity corrected. Data on top are from ATAP; bottom are from MOAFTS. ATAP= Australian Twin ADHD Project; MOAFTS=Missouri Adolescent Female Twin Study.
Source. Data summarized from Rasmussen et al. 2004.

that even modest levels of attention impairment can markedly worsen school performance (Todd et al. 2002).

In summary, in population-based samples of child and adolescent and young adult twins, we have been able to replicate the factor structure of ADHD symptoms reported from clinical and school-based samples. However, reanalysis of these data using latent-class approaches demonstrates the presence of multiple independent ADHD subtypes that are individually highly heritable, some of which are associated with academic problems. Given the family specificity of the latent-class subtyping approach, we believe that these latent-class subtypes represent more appropriate phenotypes for genetic studies than either DSM-IV-TR subtypes or continuum models.

AUTISTIC DEFICITS IN THE GENERAL POPULATION

As defined in DSM-IV-TR, autism and the related diagnoses of Asperger's disorder and pervasive developmental disorder not otherwise specified (PDD NOS) represent some of the most severe syndromes of childhood onset. These disorders are characterized by marked deficits in interpersonal social behavior (reciprocal social behavior), language and communication, and restricted/stereotypic behaviors and activities. To receive a diagnosis of autism, an individual has to have marked deficits in all three areas. A diagnosis of Asperger's disorder requires marked deficits in reciprocal social behavior and restricted/stereotypic interests and activities but no deficits in language. An individual with marked deficits in at least one of these areas but who does not meet the full criteria for autism is diagnosed with PDD NOS. An implication of this diagnostic scheme is that there are individual factors for these three symptom areas. Hence, one would anticipate being able to discern dimensions or categories of problems in each of these symptom areas that have distinct etiologies.

We initially set out to develop a new scale for measuring autistic symptoms in the school-age population by teachers and parents by collating DSM-IV and other symptom information from a variety of standard research instruments for the study of autism (Constantino et al. 2000). The goal was to develop a more convenient screening instrument for teachers and parents that required no intuition of the inner meaning of symptoms from the point of view of the child but only reporting on the severity and frequency of observed behaviors. As originally conceived, this instrument had seven symptom groupings covering all aspects of reciprocal social behavior, including language and communication and restricted stereotypic interests. As described by Constantino and colleagues (2000), the scale originally called the Social Reciprocity Scale (SRS; now renamed the Social Responsiveness Scale) has sound psychometric characteristics and can reliably discriminate typically developing schoolchildren from children with clinical cases of PDDs. In addition, there are marked group differences between mean scores for non-PDD child psychiatric patients without autism spectrum disorders versus children with autistic spectrum disorders (see Figure 3–3). When we examined the distribution of scores both in randomly identified schoolchildren and in population-based samples of child and adolescent twins (Figure 3–4), we observed that the distribution of scores was continuous up into the clinical range of severity and that 1.6% of boys and 0.6% of girls scored at or above the mean score for males with clinically ascertained PDD NOS (Constantino and Todd 2003). Factor analysis of SRS scores and cluster analysis of both those scores and Autism Diagnostic Interview–Revised data in both clinical and nonclinical samples were all highly consistent with the presence of a single factor. Moreover, in the best-fitting latent-class model, all classes had the same general shape with no evidence of discrete subtypes (Figure 3–5). These findings stand in contrast to the results for ADHD (and to our initial expectations, given assumptions from previous clinical studies), in that autistic symptoms in the general population are apparently best construed as following a continuum. The degree of communication and stereotypic symptoms were generally highly correlated with the degree of deficits in reciprocal social behavior. Put another way, there is no evidence for discrete subtypes of autistic disorders in the general population. This concept is in keeping with some previous and recent analyses of families identified through autistic probands in which deficits in family members showed no evidence of clustering of symptom subtypes or components (Pickles et al. 2000; Spiker et al. 2002).

Assuming a continuum model for underlying heritability to autism, we conducted heritability analyses of reciprocal social behavior deficits in our epidemiological twin sample (MO1 WINS). Results of these analyses are summarized in Table 3–3. For male–male twin pairs, the best-fitting genetic model included significant additive genetic effects and significant unique environmental effects without evidence for the presence of common or shared environment effects. The heritability estimate ($a^2 = 0.76$) is in keeping with previous estimates from twin studies using categorically defined autism. Interestingly, when an identical analysis was done for female–female twin pairs, a different view arose. In this case the best-fitting model had significant additive genetic,

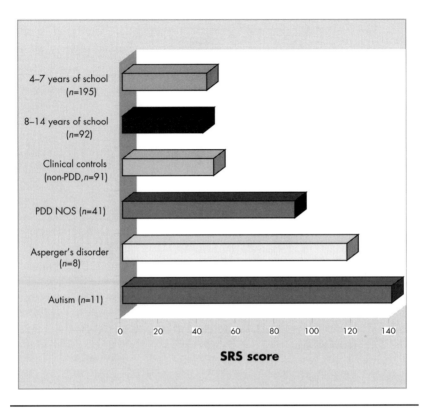

FIGURE 3-3.   Mean Social Reciprocity Scale (SRS) scores for different diagnostic groups.

Clinical control subjects include clinical cases of nonautistic spectrum diagnoses. Schoolchildren were randomly chosen by age group. PDD=pervasive developmental disorder; PDD NOS=pervasive developmental disorder not otherwise specified.

shared environment, and unique environment effects, with shared environment effects being predominant (c^2=0.44). To try to understand the significant difference in heritability estimates for boys and girls, we additionally included SRS measures from the parents of opposite-sex twin pairs in joint analyses to determine whether sex-specific genetic effects were present. We were able to rule out the presence of sex-specific genes and overall found the best-fitting model was one in which the causal (genetic and environmental) influences on autistic traits were the same for boys and girls but the magnitude of their effects differed across genders The results suggested that early environmental effects (either during gestation or early childhood) protect girls from expressing genetic

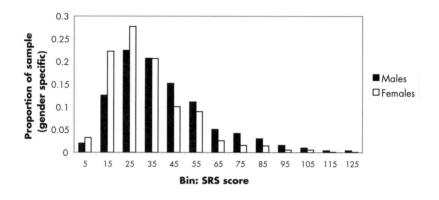

FIGURE 3–4.   Distribution of Social Reciprocity Scale (SRS) scores in an epidemiological sample of 7- to 15-year-old twins ($n=1,576$).

Note.   Bin refers to the binning of SRS scores displayed in the histogram.

Source.   Reprinted from Constantino JN, Hudziak JJ Todd RD: "Deficits in Reciprocal Social Behavior in Male Twins: Evidence for a Genetically Independent Domain of Psychopathology." *Journal of the American Academy of Child and Adolescent Psychiatry* 42:458–467, 2003. Copyright 2003, RD Todd and JN Constantino. Used with permission.

liability to social behavioral deficits (resulting in a shared environmental factor on the order of 44% for girls).

In preliminary studies, we have also measured reciprocal social behavior in parents and siblings of autistic individuals and the parents and siblings of nonautistic children. Our initial findings are that father–son correlations are much higher than other correlations within families for both clinical and nonclinical families. Again, this finding is most compatible with a continuum risk model for autistic symptoms and demonstrates the same-sex effect pattern as seen in twin samples.

In summary, in contrast to the results for ADHD, similar analyses of the clustering of samples in autistic spectrum disorders suggest that the best model of disease is a continuum model with marked sex effects. There is little current evidence to suggest separable domains of risk for the three DSM-IV-TR-defined symptom areas of autism.

INTERACTION OF ADHD AND AUTISM DOMAINS

It is frequently clinically observed that many children with an autistic spectrum disorder also have prominent problems with attention and hyperactivity and that many children with ADHD have problems with

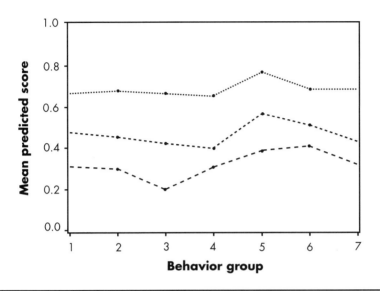

FIGURE 3–5. Latent-class analysis of Social Reciprocity Scale (SRS) data from normal schoolchildren (*n*=287).

Source. Redrawn from Constantino JN, Przybeck T, Friesen D, et al.: "Reciprocal Social Behavior in Children With and Without Pervasive Developmental Disorders." *Journal of Developmental and Behavioral Pediatrics* 21:2–11, 2000. Used with permission.

TABLE 3–3. Heritability of reciprocal social behavior deficits

Sex	Model	P^*	a^2	c^2	e^2
Male	ACE	0.31	0.76	0.00	0.24
	AE	0.48	0.76	—	0.24
	CE	0.00			
	E	0.00			
Female	ACE	0.44	0.33	0.44	0.23
	AE	0.00			
	CE	0.01			
	E	0.00			

Note. ACE=variance in a trait explained by additive genetics (A), shared environment (c), and nonshared environment (e).

*Higher value=better fit.

Source. Data summarized from Constantino and Todd 2003.

interpersonal social skills. However, in DSM-IV-TR you cannot give both diagnoses to the same child. As an initial attempt to try to characterize the possible overlap or interaction of these two domains of psychopathology, we reported on the interactions of reciprocal social behavioral deficits as measured by the SRS with attention problems as measured by the Child Behavior Checklist Attention Problem (CBCL-AP) scale in a random subset of the MOTWINS epidemiologically ascertained male twins. We did not have sufficient numbers of diagnostic interviews on this sample to allow analysis by ADHD latent class, but we were able to use the CBCL-AP scale as a proxy for inattention problems (Constantino et al. 2003).

Previous analyses had demonstrated that CBCL-AP scores are highly heritable for boys and girls in this sample (Hudziak et al. 2000). When the association between reciprocal social behavior and attention problems was analyzed by simple regression analysis of CBCL subscale scores, there was no significant association between six subscales of the CBCL and SRS values. As expected, there was a significant association between the SRS and the CBCL Social Problems subscale, because these instruments contain a number of overlapping items. However, we also observed a significant positive association between the CBCL-AP and SRS scores. Bivariate genetic analysis of these two domains demonstrated that the SRS and the CBCL-AP scale results were both highly heritable but largely genetically independent. When we tested for the influence of one scale on the other, we found significant evidence for a positive phenotypic influence of the SRS on the CBCL-AP scale but not the opposite—that is, increased deviance in reciprocal social behavior resulted in increased measures of attention problems through a nongenetic mechanism.

These results demonstrate that ADHD problems that are highly heritable (as described earlier) can be influenced by the degree of social deviance by the child. This finding may offer a natural mechanism for the observed co-occurrence of these two problem areas in clinical samples and also emphasizes the possible need for the inclusion of measures of social reciprocity in genetic studies of ADHD. We are in the process of collecting SRS data on children who have been more extensively studied for ADHD deficits so we can extend this analysis to a consideration of specific ADHD latent-class subtypes.

CONCLUSION

Population-based analyses of individual symptoms of ADHD and autism lead us to propose opposite structures for these two early-onset syndromes.

TABLE 3–4.   Conclusions from population-based studies

	ADHD	Autism
Discrete forms of disorder	+	−
Continuum disorder	−	+
Heritability	70%–90%[a]	76% male 40% female
DSM-IV-TR criteria for genetic studies	Poor	Poor
Gene × environment	+	+

Note.   ADHD=attention-deficit/hyperactivity disorder.
[a]Male and female.

For ADHD our analyses suggest that multiple genetically discrete forms of the disorder are present. Latent-class-defined categories appeared to be better phenotypes for genetic analyses than DSM-IV-TR subtypes (Table 3–4). In contrast, autistic symptoms appear to be best modeled as a continuum of severity in the general population. Heritability estimates for autism are higher for males than for females, although there appear to be no male-specific genetic factors. There may be important environmental mediating variables that protect girls from social reciprocal deficits or that amplify these deficits in boys and may be partially responsible for the consistently observed gender differences (4:1, male:female) in prevalence for all common PDDs (autistic disorder, Asperger's disorder, PDD NOS). Hence, we have found evidence for possible gene–environment interactions for subthreshold social impairments characteristic of autism spectrum conditions. We have also found evidence that these two domains of psychopathology interact to amplify ADHD symptoms through nongenetic mechanisms.

In general, whether the population-derived phenotypes will be more useful in identifying genes is yet to be demonstrated. However, in a preliminary application of this approach to ADHD, we have recently reported on the significant association of a sequence variation in the nicotinic acetylcholine alpha-4 receptor gene (*CHRNA4*) in latent-class-defined "severe inattention problems" that was not present in other DSM-IV-TR or latent-class-defined ADHD subtypes (Todd et al. 2003). In other preliminary studies we have found significant associations of dopamine receptor *DRD5* gene polymorphisms in the latent-class-defined combined ADHD subtype but not for other DSM-IV-TR or latent-class-defined ADHD subtypes. These findings, which await replication, suggest that the use of population-defined phenotypes results in identification of more genetically homogeneous forms of ADHD. Similar studies have not been conducted for autism. We note, however, that the application of these approaches to existing genetic studies of autism would be feasible and relatively inexpensive using newly established methodologies for assessment of symptoms.

REFERENCES

American Psychiatric Association: Diagnostic and Statistical Manual of Mental Disorders, 4th Edition. Washington, DC, American Psychiatric Association, 1994

American Psychiatric Association: Diagnostic and Statistical Manual of Mental Disorders, 4th Edition, Text Revision. Washington, DC, American Psychiatric Association, 2000

Constantino JN, Todd RD: Autistic traits in the general population: a twin study. Arch Gen Psychiatry 60:524–530, 2003

Constantino JN, Przybeck T, Friesen D, et al: Reciprocal social behavior in children with and without pervasive developmental disorders. J Dev Behav Pediatr 21:2–11, 2000

Constantino JN, Hudziak JJ, Todd RD: Deficits in reciprocal social behavior in male twins: evidence for a genetically independent domain of psychopathology. J Am Acad Child Adolesc Psychiatry 42:458–467, 2003

Helzer JE, Hudziak JJ: Defining Psychopathology in the 21st Century: DSM-V and Beyond. Washington, DC, American Psychiatric Publishing, 2002

Hudziak JJ, Heath AC, Madden PF, et al: Latent class and factor analysis of DSM-IV ADHD: a twin study of female adolescents. J Am Acad Child Adolesc Psychiatry 37:848–857, 1998

Hudziak JJ, Rudiger LP, Neale MC, et al: A twin study of inattentive, aggressive, and anxious/depressed behaviors. J Am Acad Child Adolesc Psychiatry 39:469–476, 2000

Neuman RJ, Todd RD, Heath AC, et al: Evaluation of ADHD typology in three contrasting samples: a latent class approach. J Am Acad Child Adolesc Psychiatry 38:25–33, 1999

Pickles A, Starr E, Kazak S, et al: Variable expression of the autism broader phenotype: findings from extended pedigrees. J Child Psychol Psychiatry 41:491–502, 2000

Rasmussen ER, Neuman RJ, Heath AC, et al: Replication of the latent class structure of attention-deficit/hyperactivity disorder (ADHD) subtypes in a sample of Australian twins. J Child Psychol Psychiatry 43:1018–1028, 2002

Rasmussen ER, Neuman RJ, Heath AC, et al: Familial clustering of latent class and DSM-IV defined attention-deficit/hyperactivity disorder subtypes. J Child Psychol Psychiatry 45:589–598, 2004

Spiker D, Lotspeich LJ, Dimiceli S, et al: Behavioral phenotypic variation in autism multiplex families: evidence for a continuous severity gradient. Am J Med Genet 114:129–136, 2002

Todd RD: Genetic Contributions to Early Onset Psychopathology. Philadelphia, PA, WB Saunders, 2001

Todd RD, Rasmussen ER, Neuman RJ, et al: Familiality and heritability of subtypes of attention deficit hyperactivity disorder in a population sample of adolescent female twins. Am J Psychiatry 158:1891–1898, 2001

Todd RD, Sitdhiraksa N, Reich W, et al: Discrimination of DSM-IV and latent class attention deficit/hyperactivity disorder subtypes by educational and cognitive performance in a population based sample of child and adolescent twins. J Am Acad Child Adolesc Psychiatry 41:820–828, 2002

Todd RD, Lobos EA, Sun LW, et al: Mutational analysis of the nicotinic acetylcholine receptor alpha 4 subunit gene in attention deficit/hyperactivity disorder: evidence for association of an intronic polymorphism with attention problems. Mol Psychiatry 8:103–108, 2003

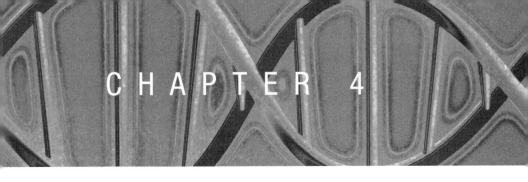

CHAPTER 4

Genetic Risk Factors for Late-Onset Alzheimer's Disease

Petra Nowotny, Ph.D.

Scott Smemo, B.A.

Alison M. Goate, D.Phil.

Alzheimer's disease (AD) is a complex neurodegenerative disorder characterized by gradual onset and progression of memory loss combined with deficits in executive functioning, language, visuospatial abilities, personality, behavior, and self-care. Neuropathological evaluation of AD cases at autopsy reveals the presence of large numbers of neurofibrillary tangles and senile plaques. Neurofibrillary tangles are intracellular inclusions composed of polymerized hyperphosphorylated tau, and senile plaques are extracellular aggregates of insoluble β-amyloid (Aβ). Aβ is a 39- to 43–amino acid peptide generated by proteolytic cleavage of the amyloid precursor protein (APP) by β- and γ-secretases. Ninety percent of soluble Aβ is A_{40}, whereas most of the remaining 10% of soluble Aβ is composed of longer, more fibrillogenic peptides.

It is estimated that 4 million people in the United States have AD, resulting in 100,000 deaths per year. The risk of developing AD increases substantially with age: 1%–5% of the population older than 65 years has

AD, whereas 20%–40% of those older than 85 years have AD (Small et al. 1997). As a result, the vast majority of AD patients have an onset of disease after age 65 (late-onset AD), whereas only 2%–3% have onset before 65 (early-onset AD; Ott et al. 1995). All AD patients, regardless of age at onset, develop similar cognitive impairments and pathological lesions in the brain.

GENETICS OF ALZHEIMER'S DISEASE

There are two forms of AD: *familial AD,* in which the disease is transmitted as an autosomal dominant trait, and *sporadic* AD, which shows modest familial clustering and probably results from the synergistic action of genetic and environmental factors. Familial AD accounts for less than 1% of AD cases and usually has an age at onset younger than 65 years. Sporadic AD can have an early (younger than 60 years) or late (older than 60 years) age at onset. Familial AD does not appear to be clinically or neuropathologically different from the more common sporadic form of AD, except that it generally has an earlier age at onset.

Familial AD is caused by autosomal dominant mutations in one of three genes that encode APP (Goate et al. 1991; Levy-Lahad et al. 1995), presenilin 1 (*PS1*; Sherrington et al. 1995), and presenilin 2 (*PS2*; Levy-Lahad et al. 1995; Rogaev et al. 1995). Mutations in each of these genes result in higher $A\beta_{42}$ levels (Scheuner et al. 1996). This observation led to the suggestion that $A\beta$ metabolism is central to the disease process, at least in familial AD cases. Indeed, mice overexpressing a human *APP* transgene carrying a familial AD mutation develop age-dependent $A\beta$ deposition in the brain (Games et al. 1995; Hsiao 1995). Age at onset of the disease appears to be largely determined by the mutation. In general, *PS1* mutations are associated with the earliest age at onset of the disease (25–60 years), whereas *PS2* mutations lead to a somewhat later and more variable age at onset.

For the majority of AD cases, no single gene has been found that is sufficient to cause disease. However, epidemiological studies have identified age (most AD patients have an age at onset greater than 65 years) and family history (40% have one or more affected first-degree relatives; van Duijn et al. 1991) as significant risk factors in multiple studies. Head injury with loss of consciousness appears to be an environmental risk factor for disease that shows an interaction with the apolipoprotein E (*APOE*) genotype, the only known genetic risk factor for AD. Years of education, use of NSAIDS, and use of statins have all been suggested as possible protective factors.

APOLIPOPROTEIN E

Most Aβ found in cerebrospinal fluid and in the brain is bound to APOE-containing particles. It is believed that APOE plays a role in the clearance of Aβ. The *APOE* gene is located in a region on chromosome 19 that had been linked to disease in late-onset AD families (Strittmatter et al. 1993). *APOE* has three common alleles, ε2, ε3, and ε4, generated by cysteine/arginine substitutions at two polymorphic sites at codons 112 and 158. Inheriting one or two ε4 alleles increases the risk of developing AD and results in an earlier mean age at onset in comparison to individuals with ε2 or ε3 alleles (Corder et al. 1993). There is a dose-dependent increase in risk for disease (Corder et al. 1993; Frisoni et al. 1995). One ε4 allele increases the risk of developing AD two- to fivefold, and two alleles increase the risk five- to tenfold or more (Bertram and Tanzi 2001). In contrast, the ε2 allele seems to delay the age at onset of the disease (Corder et al. 1994) and reduce risk for disease. Individuals with an ε4 allele also have a higher plaque burden at autopsy (Schmechel et al. 1993).

In contrast to all other association-based findings in AD, the association with ε4 has been consistently replicated in a large number of studies across many ethnic groups and has also been found in early-onset sporadic AD (Farrer et al. 1997). The association between *APOE* ε4 and AD is weaker among African-Americans (odds ratio [OR]=1.1 for ε3/ε4; OR= 5.7 for ε4/ε4) and Hispanics (OR=2.2 for ε3/ε4; OR=2.2 for ε4/ε4) but stronger in the Japanese population (OR=5.6 for ε3/ε4; OR= 33.1 for ε4/ε4) compared with Caucasians (OR 3.2=ε3/ε4; OR=14.9 for ε4/ε4) (Farrer et al. 1997).

Crosses between *APOE*[-/-] mice and *APP* transgenic mice have demonstrated that *APOE* is necessary for generation of fibrillar Aβ, thioflavin S–positive amyloid deposition, and neuritic plaque formation (Bales et al. 1997). Furthermore, introduction of human *APOE* alleles into these crosses (*APPV717F:APOE*[-/-]*:APOE2/3/4*) demonstrates that the human ε4 allele leads to earlier generation of thioflavin S–positive plaques and neuritic plaques than the ε3 allele (Holtzman et al. 2000). Animals expressing human *APOE* ε2 do not develop thioflavin S–positive plaques.

Genetic and transgenic studies thus show that both familial AD mutations and *APOE* alleles influence risk for disease through Aβ-dependent mechanisms. If common pathogenic pathways are involved, *APOE* alleles might be expected to also modulate age at onset in familial AD families. However, most studies have suggested that there is little variation in age at onset within familial AD kindreds, with most variation being between families carrying different familial AD mutations.

Earlier studies in a kindred with an *APP* mutation (V717I) reported that the presence of an ε4 allele was associated with an earlier age at onset within the family, whereas the presence of an ε2 allele delayed the age at onset (Sorbi et al. 1995; St. George-Hyslop et al. 1994). This epistatic effect has not been observed with other *APP* or *PS* mutations (Laws et al. 2003). However, a major problem in addressing this issue is the small number of individuals available from single families, making statistical analysis impossible. In studies using individuals from different families carrying different mutations, the epistatic effect of *APOE* alleles might be obscured by the larger differences in age at onset associated with different familial AD mutations.

To rigorously address the effect of *APOE* alleles on age at onset, we examined a large Colombian kindred carrying the E280A mutation in *PS1*. More than 20 nuclear families have been reported from the same region of Colombia that carry the same mutation. Genealogical and haplotype analyses demonstrate that there is a founder effect in this population. The common ancestor is believed to have emigrated from Spain to Colombia 200 to 300 years ago; thus, each nuclear family is distantly related to the other nuclear families. The age at onset in these kindreds is broad (35–65 years), suggesting that genetic or environmental risk factors may modify age at onset. Survival analysis was used to examine time to age at onset in E280A carriers with or without *APOE* ε4 alleles. A total of 109 individuals carrying the E280A mutation were available for this study: 57 subjects who remained asymptomatic throughout the study period and 52 individuals who received a diagnosis of probable AD at or before their last visit. The log-rank test showed a statistically significant difference ($P=0.045$) among the two survival functions of time to AD onset in the two groups. Kindred members with an *APOE* ε4 allele were more likely to develop AD at an earlier age than were members without an *APOE* ε4 allele (Pastor et al. 2003). Furthermore, individuals with an *APOE* ε2 allele developed the disease at a later age, although the difference in age at onset was not statistically significant, most likely because of the small number of individuals carrying *APOE* ε2 alleles. These results support the hypothesis that there is a single common disease pathway that involves Aβ in familial and sporadic AD, suggesting both forms could be responsive to anti-Aβ therapies.

SEARCH FOR NEW ALZHEIMER'S DISEASE RISK GENES

The four known genes (*APP, PS1, PS2,* and *APOE*) account for only 20%–50% of the total heritability of AD. Indeed, more than half of all AD cases carry none of these risk factors (Saunders 2000). Segregation analysis in 75 late-onset AD families (treating AD as a quantitative locus based on age at onset) not only detected the known effects of the *APOE* ε4 and ε2 alleles but also found evidence for four additional loci that make a contribution to age at onset comparable in magnitude to *APOE* and one locus that had a much greater effect on age at onset than did *APOE* (Warwick Daw et al. 2000).

To look for other genetic risk factors, several groups performed genomewide screens in affected sibling pairs or late-onset AD families (Blacker et al. 2003; Kehoe et al. 1999; Myers et al. 2002; Pericak-Vance et al. 1997). The earliest used a two-stage design, first genotyping markers at 10-cM intervals in late-onset AD families and then examining regions with a LOD score greater than 1 or a *P* value less than 0.05 in an additional 38 families (Pericak-Vance et al. 1997). They found evidence of linkage to chromosomes 4, 6, 12 and 20, with the strongest result on chromosome 12 (multipoint LOD score [MLS]=3.9). More recently, this group rescreened the entire genome in 466 families using parametric and nonparametric analyses (Pericak-Vance et al. 2000). The most significant MLS, 4.3, in this screen was on chromosome 9. Our own group also used a two-stage design, first genotyping 237 markers spaced at approximately 20-cM intervals in 292 late-onset AD–affected sibling pairs (Kehoe et al. 1999), then following up regions with an MLS greater than 1 with a denser marker set in 450 sibling pairs (Myers et al. 2002). In stage 1, 16 regions on chromosomes 1 (two peaks), 5, 6, 9 (two peaks), 10, 12 (two peaks), 13, 14, 19, 21, and X (two peaks) gave a LOD score greater than 1. The highest LOD scores on chromosome 1 (MLS=2.67), 9 (MLS= 2.38), 10 (MLS=2.27), and 19 (MLS=1.79) fulfill the criteria of "suggestive" linkage. Ten regions maintained an MLS greater than 1 in stage 2: chromosomes 1, 5, 6, 9, (two peaks), 10, 12, 19, 21, and X. The most significant evidence for linkage was on chromosome 10, with an MLS of 3.9 between the markers D10S1227 and D10DS1225. The linkage to chromosome 10 was not affected by *APOE* genotype.

Blacker et al. (2003) reported a 9-cM genome screen of 437 families with a highly significant peak on chromosome 19q13 (probably *APOE*) and 12 additional regions on 1q23, 3p26, 4q32, 5p14, 6p21, 6p27, 9q22, 10q24, 11q25, 14q22, 15q26, and 21q22 with MLS greater than 2.2 (suggestive linkage).

In addition to these studies, Farrer et al. (2003) performed a genomewide association study in an inbred Israeli-Arab community with a high prevalence of AD. Strong evidence for association was observed with markers on chromosomes 2, 9, 10, and 12. All of these regions except the locus on chromosome 2 have been implicated in risk for late-onset AD in outbred populations.

Additional evidence for an AD locus on chromosome 10 has come from a quantitative trait locus study using plasma Aβ levels as the trait (Ertekin-Taner et al. 2000). For this linkage study, families were identified in which high plasma Aβ levels segregated as a heritable trait. Microsatellite markers were genotyped on chromosomes 1, 5, 9, 10, and 19, as a follow-up to results from Kehoe et al. (1999). The most significant evidence for linkage (MLS=3.9) was in the 80-cM region of chromosome 10 between markers D10S1227 and D10S1211, in agreement with the region described by Myers et al. (2000).

Another region on chromosome 10 (~115–130 cM) was identified in a linkage study in 435 families with six markers around insulin-degrading enzyme (MLS=3.4; Bertram et al. 2000). To identify genes influencing age at onset in AD and Parkinson's disease, Li et al. (2002) performed a genome screen . For AD, the age at onset effect of *APOE* was confirmed and, in addition, Li et al. found linkage to a region on chromosome 10 between D10S1239 and D101237, which is close to the region identified by Bertram et al. (2000).

Other studies (Rogaeva et al. 1998; Wu et al. 1998) confirmed the linkage finding on chromosome 12 (Pericak-Vance et al. 1997), although the locations of their linkage peaks are not identical to those in the original report. In 2000 Pericak-Vance's group refined the original linkage region by genotyping more markers (Scott et al. 2000).

Additional evidence for linkage to chromosome 12p was found in a study using 35 markers and 79 Caribbean Hispanic families with AD at two sites (Mayeux et al. 2002). The two-point LOD scores were 3.15 at D12S1623 and 1.43 at D12S1042, but the linkage varied with age at onset and presence or absence of the *APOE* ε4 allele.

In summary, all genome screens have shown linkage to chromosome 19 (*APOE*). Other regions, which appear to replicate between studies, are on chromosomes 9, 10, and 12, although the precise location of the peak evidence of linkage varies markedly between studies. Table 4–1 summarizes the results of genome screens and linkage studies.

CANDIDATE GENES

A large number of candidate genes—for example, genes that are involved in Aβ production, aggregation, degradation, and clearance; lipid-metabolism; or inflammation—have been evaluated in AD association and linkage studies because of the known biology of the disease. Some of these

TABLE 4–1. Results of genome screens and linkage studies

Study	Chromosome[a]	Location[b]	Results[c]
Pericak-Vance et al. 1997[d]	4, 6, **12**, 20	30	MLS: 3.9
Wu et al. 1998	12	12	MLS: 1.9
Rogaeva et al. 1998	12	54	NPLS: 3.5
Zubenko et al. 1998[d]	1, 10, 12, 19, X		
Kehoe et al. 1999[d]	**1**, 5, **9, 10**, 12, 14, **19**, 21		All MLS: ~2
Pericak-Vance et al. 2000[d]	**9**	26, 137	MLS: 4.3, 2.0
Bertram et al. 2000	**10**	99	TLS: 3.3, 3.4
Ertekin-Taner et al. 2000	**10**	67	MLS: 3.9
Mayeux et al. 2002	12	7, 24	TLS : 3.15, 1.43
Myers et al. 2002[d]	1, 5, 6, 9, **10**, 12, 19, 21, X	67	MLS: 3.9
Blacker et al. 2003[d]	1, 3, 4, 5, 6, 9, 10, 11, 14, 15, 21		All MLS: ≥ 2.2
Farrer et al. 2003[d]	2, 9, 10, 12		

Note. MLS=multipoint LOD score; NPLS=nonparametric linkage score; TLS=two-point LOD score.
[a]The strongest finding is printed in bold.
[b]Approximate location for the strongest finding, in megabases from the telomere of the p arm of the chromosome.
[c]Result is for the strongest finding.
[d]These studies are genomewide screens.

genes have been located in chromosomal regions with evidence for linkage, making them positional and biological candidate genes. The two chromosomal regions that have been analyzed most extensively are on chromosomes 10 and 12. On chromosome 10 both positive and negative association studies have been reported for insulin-degrading enzyme and for urokinase-type plasminogen activator (Abraham et al. 2001; Bertram et al. 2000; Boussaha et al. 2002; Myers et al. 2004). Both of these proteins have been implicated in Aβ degradation, making them strong biological candidate genes (McDermott and Gibson 1997; Qiu et al. 1998; Vekrellis et al. 2000). The gene encoding α-T-catenin, *CTNNA3*, is also positioned within the linkage region on chromosome 10 (Myers et al. 2000), close to D10S1211. It is expressed in brain, inhibits Wnt signaling, and is therefore a good functional and positional candidate. Genotyping several single nucleotide polymorphisms in this gene did not show any association with the disease (Busby et al. 2004). Similarly, the genes encoding α_2-macroglobulin and the low-density lipoprotein receptor–related protein on chromosome 12 have both been extensively analyzed (Blacker et al. 1998; Kang et al. 1997; Liao et al. 1998). These two proteins have been implicated in Aβ clearance (Hyman et al. 2000; Kang et al. 2000); however, genetic association studies have not consistently observed an effect on risk for disease (Fallin et al. 1997; Koster et al. 2000).

CONCLUSION

In the Mendelian forms of AD, mutations in three genes have been shown to cause the disease by increasing the production of the longer Aβ species, Aβ_{42}, which forms aggregates easily. The only known genetic risk factor for late-onset AD identified so far is *APOE*, which facilitates Aβ fibril formation. *APOE* also reduces the age at onset of disease in both familial AD and sporadic early and late-onset AD.

Linkage studies have identified regions on chromosomes 9, 10, and 12 that are associated with late-onset AD in multiple studies. Unfortunately, these linkage peaks span tens of megabases containing hundreds of candidate genes. However, two key genomics developments will speed the process of identifying the specific genes and their variants that modify the risk for developing AD: the data generated by the Human Genome Project and the continuing refinement of haplotype block maps.

REFERENCES

Abraham R, Myers A, Wavrant-DeVrieze F, et al: Substantial linkage disequilibrium across the insulin-degrading enzyme locus but no association with late-onset Alzheimer's disease. Hum Genet 109:646–652, 2001

Bales KR, Verina T, Dodel RC, et al: Lack of apolipoprotein E dramatically reduces amyloid beta-peptide deposition. Nat Genet 17:263–264, 1997

Bertram L, Tanzi RE: Dancing in the dark? The status of late-onset Alzheimer's disease genetics. J Mol Neurosci 17:127–136, 2001

Bertram L, Blacker D, Mullin K, et al: Evidence for genetic linkage of Alzheimer's disease to chromosome 10q. Science 290:2302–2303, 2000

Blacker D, Wilcox MA, Laird NM, et al: Alpha-2 macroglobulin is genetically associated with Alzheimer disease. Nat Genet 19:357–360, 1998

Blacker D, Bertram L, Saunders AJ, et al: Results of a high-resolution genome screen of 437 Alzheimer's disease families. Hum Mol Genet 12:23–32, 2003

Boussaha M, Hannequin D, Verpillat P, et al: Polymorphisms of insulin degrading enzyme gene are not associated with Alzheimer's disease. Neurosci Lett 329:121–123, 2002

Busby V, Goossens S, Nowotny P, et al: Alpha-T-catenin is expressed in human brain and interacts with the Wnt signaling pathway but is not responsible for linkage to chromosome 10 in Alzheimer's disease. Neuromolecular Med 5:133–146, 2004

Corder EH, Saunders AM, Strittmatter WJ, et al: Gene dose of apolipoprotein E type 4 allele and the risk of Alzheimer's disease in late onset families. Science 261:921–923, 1993

Corder EH, Saunders AM, Risch NJ, et al: Protective effect of apolipoprotein E type 2 allele for late onset Alzheimer disease. Nat Genet 7:180–184, 1994

Ertekin-Taner N, Graff-Radford N, Younkin LH, et al: Linkage of plasma Aβ42 to a quantitative locus on chromosome 10 in late-onset Alzheimer's disease pedigrees. Science 290:2303–2304, 2000

Fallin D, Kundtz A, Town T, et al: No association between the low density lipoprotein receptor-related protein (LRP) gene and late-onset Alzheimer's disease in a community-based sample. Neurosci Lett 233:145–147, 1997

Farrer LA, Cupples LA, Haines JL, et al: Effects of age, sex, and ethnicity on the association between apolipoprotein E genotype and Alzheimer disease: a meta-analysis. APOE and Alzheimer Disease Meta Analysis Consortium. JAMA 278:1349–1356, 1997

Farrer LA, Bowirrat A, Friedland RP, et al: Identification of multiple loci for Alzheimer disease in a consanguineous Israeli-Arab community. Hum Mol Genet 12:415–422, 2003

Frisoni GB, Govoni S, Geroldi C, et al: Gene dose of the epsilon 4 allele of apolipoprotein E and disease progression in sporadic late-onset Alzheimer's disease. Ann Neurol 37:596–604, 1995

Games D, Adams D, Alessandrini R, et al: Alzheimer-type neuropathology in transgenic mice overexpressing V717F beta-amyloid precursor protein. Nature 373:523–527, 1995

Goate A, Chartier-Harlin MC, Mullan M, et al: Segregation of a missense mutation in the amyloid precursor protein gene with familial Alzheimer's disease. Nature 349:704–706, 1991

Holtzman DM, Bales KR, Tenkova T, et al: Apolipoprotein E isoform-dependent amyloid deposition and neuritic degeneration in a mouse model of Alzheimer's disease. Proc Natl Acad Sci U S A 97:2892–2897, 2000

Hsiao KK: Understanding the biology of beta-amyloid precursor proteins in transgenic mice. Neurobiol Aging 16:705–706, 1995

Hyman BT, Strickland D, Rebeck GW: Role of the low-density lipoprotein receptor-related protein in beta-amyloid metabolism and Alzheimer disease. Arch Neurol 57:646–650, 2000

Kang DE, Saitoh T, Chen X, et al: Genetic association of the low-density lipoprotein receptor-related protein gene (LRP), an apolipoprotein E receptor, with late-onset Alzheimer's disease. Neurology 49:56–61, 1997

Kang DE, Pietrzik CU, Baum L, et al: Modulation of amyloid beta-protein clearance and Alzheimer's disease susceptibility by the LDL receptor-related protein pathway. J Clin Invest 106:1159–1166, 2000

Kehoe P, Wavrant-De Vrieze F, Crook R, et al: A full genome scan for late onset Alzheimer's disease. Hum Mol Genet 8:237–245, 1999

Koster MN, Dermaut B, Cruts M, et al: The alpha2-macroglobulin gene in AD: a population-based study and meta-analysis. Neurology 55:678–684, 2000

Laws SM, Hone E, Gandy S, et al: Expanding the association between the APOE gene and the risk of Alzheimer's disease: possible roles for APOE promoter polymorphisms and alterations in APOE transcription. J Neurochem 84: 1215–1236, 2003

Levy-Lahad E, Wasco W, Poorkaj P, et al: Candidate gene for the chromosome 1 familial Alzheimer's disease locus. Science 269:973–977, 1995

Li YJ, Scott WK, Hedges DJ, et al: Age at onset in two common neurodegenerative diseases is genetically controlled. Am J Hum Genet 70:985–993, 2002

Liao A, Nitsch RM, Greenberg SM, et al: Genetic association of an alpha2-macroglobulin (Val1000lle) polymorphism and Alzheimer's disease. Hum Mol Genet 7:1953–1956, 1998

Mayeux R, Lee JH, Romas SN, et al: Chromosome-12 mapping of late-onset Alzheimer disease among Caribbean Hispanics. Am J Hum Genet 70:237–243, 2002

McDermott J, Gibson A: Degradation of Alzheimer's beta-amyloid protein by human and rat brain peptidases: involvement of insulin-degrading enzyme. Neurochem Res 22:49–56, 1997

Myers A, Holmans P, Marshall H, et al: Susceptibility locus for Alzheimer's disease on chromosome 10. Science 290:2304–2305, 2000

Myers A, Wavrant De-Vrieze F, Holmans P, et al: Full genome screen for Alzheimer disease: stage II analysis. Am J Med Genet 114:235–244, 2002

Myers A, Marshall H, Holmans P, et al: Variation in the urokinase-plasminogen activator gene does not explain the chromosome 10 linkage signal for later onset AD. Am J Med Genet B Neuropsychiatr Genet 124:29–37, 2004

Ott A, Breteler MM, van Harskamp F, et al: Prevalence of Alzheimer's disease and vascular dementia: association with education. The Rotterdam Study. BMJ 310:970–973, 1995

Pastor P, Roe C, Villegas A, et al: APOE ε4 modifies age of onset in a large E280A PS1 Alzheimer's disease kindred. Ann Neurol 54:163–169, 2003

Pericak-Vance MA, Bass MP, Yamaoka LH, et al: Complete genomic screen in late-onset familial Alzheimer disease: evidence for a new locus on chromosome 12. JAMA 278:1237–1241, 1997

Pericak-Vance MA, Grubber J, Bailey LR, et al: Identification of novel genes in late-onset Alzheimer's disease. Exp Gerontol 35:1343–1352, 2000

Qiu WQ, Walsh DM, Ye Z, et al: Insulin-degrading enzyme regulates extracellular levels of amyloid beta-protein by degradation. J Biol Chem 273:32730–32738, 1998

Rogaev EI, Sherrington R, Rogaeva EA, et al: Familial Alzheimer's disease in kindreds with missense mutations in a gene on chromosome 1 related to the Alzheimer's disease type 3 gene. Nature 376:775–778, 1995

Rogaeva E, Premkumar S, Song Y, et al: Evidence for an Alzheimer disease susceptibility locus on chromosome 12 and for further locus heterogeneity. JAMA 280:614–618, 1998

Saunders AM: Apolipoprotein E and Alzheimer disease: an update on genetic and functional analyses. J Neuropathol Exp Neurol 59:751–758, 2000

Scheuner D, Eckman C, Jensen M, et al: Secreted amyloid beta-protein similar to that in the senile plaques of Alzheimer's disease is increased in vivo by the presenilin 1 and 2 and APP mutations linked to familial Alzheimer's disease. Nat Med 2:864–870, 1996

Schmechel DE, Saunders AM, Strittmatter WJ, et al: Increased amyloid beta-peptide deposition in cerebral cortex as a consequence of apolipoprotein E genotype in late-onset Alzheimer disease. Proc Natl Acad Sci U S A 90:9649–9653, 1993

Scott WK, Grubber JM, Conneally PM, et al: Fine mapping of the chromosome 12 late-onset Alzheimer disease locus: potential genetic and phenotypic heterogeneity. Am J Hum Genet 66:922–932, 2000

Sherrington R, Rogaev EI, Liang Y, et al: Cloning of a gene bearing missense mutations in early onset familial Alzheimer's disease. Nature 375:754–760, 1995

Small GW, Rabins PV, Barry PP, et al: Diagnosis and treatment of Alzheimer disease and related disorders: consensus statement of the American Association for Geriatric Psychiatry, the Alzheimer's Association, and the American Geriatrics Society. JAMA 278:1363–1371, 1997

Sorbi S, Nacmias B, Forleo P, et al: Epistatic effect of APP717 mutation and apolipoprotein E genotype in familial Alzheimer's disease. Ann Neurol 38:124–127, 1995

St. George-Hyslop P, McLachlan DC, Tsuda T, et al: Alzheimer's disease and possible gene interaction. Science 263:537, 1994

Strittmatter WJ, Saunders AM, Schmechel D, et al: Apolipoprotein E: high-avidity binding to beta-amyloid and increased frequency of type 4 allele in late-onset familial Alzheimer disease. Proc Natl Acad Sci U S A 90:1977–1981, 1993

van Duijn CM, Clayton D, Chandra V, et al: Familial aggregation of Alzheimer's disease and related disorders: a collaborative re-analysis of case-control studies. EURODEM Risk Factors Research Group. Int J Epidemiol 20(suppl): S13–S20, 1991

Vekrellis K, Ye Z, Qiu WQ, et al: Neurons regulate extracellular levels of amyloid beta-protein via proteolysis by insulin-degrading enzyme. J Neurosci 20:1657–1665, 2000

Warwick Daw E, Payami H, Nemens EJ, et al: The number of trait loci in late-onset Alzheimer disease. Am J Hum Genet 66:196–204, 2000

Wu WS, Holmans P, Wavrant-DeVrieze F, et al: Genetic studies on chromosome 12 in late-onset Alzheimer disease. JAMA 280:619–622, 1998

Zubenko GS, Hughes HB, Stiffler JS, et al: A genome survey for novel Alzheimer disease risk loci: results at 10-cM resolution. Genomics 50:121–128, 1998

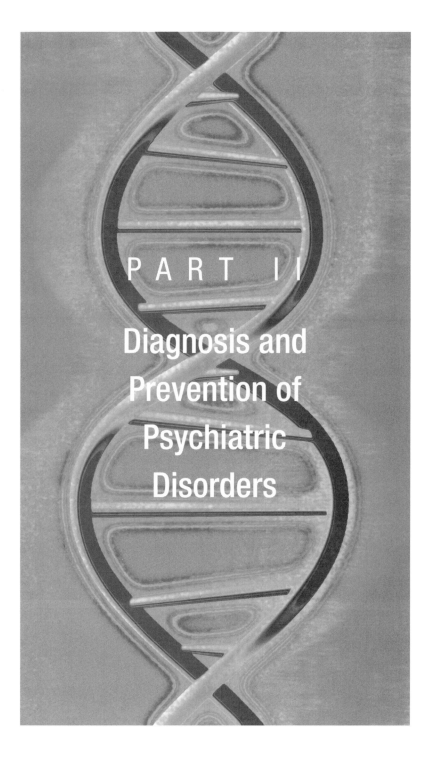

PART II

Diagnosis and
Prevention of
Psychiatric
Disorders

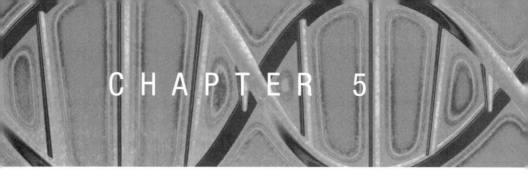

CHAPTER 5

Are There Phenotype Problems?

Peter McGuffin, M.B., Ph.D.

Anne E. Farmer, M.D.

PROBLEMS OR PUZZLES?

One of the most informative but least likely bestsellers in the literary charts of the United Kingdom of the past few years was Edmonds and Eidinow's (2001) account of the antecedents and outcome of a heated 10-minute argument between two famous twentieth-century British philosophers, Sir Karl Popper and Ludwig Wittgenstein. The argument occurred in a small seminar room in Cambridge University in October 1946 and culminated in the host, Wittgenstein, angrily picking up a poker from the fireplace and brandishing it at Popper, his visiting speaker from the London School of Economics. The reason for Wittgenstein's wrath was Popper's assertion, made clear at the very outset of his talk entitled "Are There Philosophical Problems?," that the answer was an emphatic "yes." This was a direct challenge to Wittgenstein's position that traditional philosophical problems can all be reduced to purely linguistic puzzles. The debate ended when Wittgenstein, poker in hand, challenged Popper to give him an example of a moral rule. It is said that Popper replied, "Not to threaten visiting lecturers with pokers," upon which Wittgenstein, in high dudgeon, stormed out, throwing the poker down behind him.

What does this vignette, amusing though it may be, have to do with the phenotypic problem in psychiatry? The answer is that it illustrates a polarization of philosophical views that has an uncanny parallel with the views of psychiatric experts on diagnosis and classification. On the one hand there are those who believe that the sophisticated word play of DSM-IV-TR (American Psychiatric Association 2000) has reduced the problems of psychiatric diagnosis to a series of linguistic puzzles that will eventually be solved with more of the same in DSM-V or DSM-VI and those who (like ourselves) believe that although we have come a long way, we are still faced with major phenotypic problems. We therefore, in essence, take the Popperian view and, following Popper, would advocate that the way to grapple with phenotypic problems is by a process of conjecture and refutation.

The core phenotypic problems remain the classic ones inherent in all attempts to measure psychopathology (Farmer et al. 2002)—namely, how do we achieve reliability? Once we have achieved reliability, how can we ensure that phenotypes are valid? What is the utility of the systems we are using? Finally, are we in reality dealing with discrete categories or is psychopathology always best considered in terms of dimensions? Let us start with reliability.

THE TWO ERAS OF DIAGNOSTIC RELIABILITY

In considering reliability of diagnosis, the history of psychiatry can be divided into two eras. The first era, a very long one that preceded the introduction and widespread acceptance of modern explicit criteria (before the 1970s), we can call the *before operational criteria* era, and the second, a much shorter period, we can call the *after operational criteria* era (1972 to present). The problems of diagnostic unreliability in the former era were well documented by authors in the United States in the 1960s (e.g., Beck et al. 1962; Kramer 1961), but the story began long before that and is well illustrated by the divergence of European and American views on the diagnosis of psychosis as well as by similar divergences within the United States.

For much of the middle part of the twentieth century, American psychiatry tended to follow a Bleulerian view of psychosis and took a more psychoanalytically influenced approach to psychopathology than was generally the case in Europe (Farmer et al. 2002). A further important ingredient in American psychiatry was the view put forward by Adolph Meyer that differences in subjective experiences and presentation of symptoms between individuals were as large and important as the similarity within the diagnostic groups. This teaching led to many of the categories in the first version of the American Psychiatric Association's *Diagnostic and Statistical Manual: Mental Disorders* (DSM-I; American Psychiatric Association 1952) being called "reaction types" rather than disorders. However, the trends in diagnostic practice in the United States were far from uniform, with some clinicians taking a much more Kraepelinian view. This led to substantial differences in admission rates for categories such as schizophrenia in different states. Furthermore the era before operational criteria was characterized by even larger transatlantic differences. In particular, the observation that schizophrenia was many times more common (as judged by first admission rates) in New York than in London, England (Kramer 1961) led to the U.S./U.K. Diagnostic Project (Cooper et al. 1972).

In this study, teams in London and at the New York Psychiatric Institute used a standardized interviewing method (including an early version of the Present State Examination; Wing et al. 1974) and a consensus clinical diagnosis between at least two project psychiatrists to arrive at a project diagnosis. Later, one of the ways of assessing the consistency of diagnostic habits of project psychiatrists was to check their diagnoses against a computer program, DIAGNO, devised by Dr. Robert Spitzer. The project diagnoses were then compared with local hospital diagnoses in each case. Although the hospital diagnoses assigned by local psychiatrists showed the familiar national differences between the rates of schizophrenia and manic-depressive (now known as bipolar) disorder in each site, a project diagnosis showed similar rates of diagnostic categories in the two cities. In short, a structured interview and an extended diagnostic procedure markedly improved diagnostic agreement.

Subsequently and independently, the World Health Organization mounted a wider investigation to examine cross-national diagnostic practices in a range of countries, the International Pilot Study of Schizophrenia (IPSS; World Health Organization 1973). The study included 1,200 patients in nine countries: the United States, the former U.S.S.R., United Kingdom, Denmark, Formosa (now Taiwan), Nigeria, Czechoslovakia (now the Czech Republic and Slovakia), Columbia, and India. The IPSS and the U.S./U.K. Diagnostic Project overlapped in time and in the methods used. Again each patient received a clinical diagnosis via a local psychiatrist and a project diagnosis using a semistructured interview, the Present State Examination. Indeed, the project psychiatrists from the U.S./U.K. project helped train the principal investigators from the nine IPSS sites in the use of the Present State Examination. There were discrepancies between the project diagnosis and the clinical diagnosis not just in the United States but also in the U.S.S.R., where the concept of schizophrenia had been broadened by a different set of forces. This included Snezhnevsky's concept of "sluggish schizophrenia," a diagnosis that required no positive psychotic symptoms and included individuals with socially or politically unconventional ideas. Fortunately the project diagnosis broadly showed a similar rate of schizophrenia across the nine centers. Thus reliability was achieved by taking an approach that combined a standardized interview with a computer diagnosis that essentially required that diagnoses were formulated as a set of explicit algorithms. The study therefore represented a major step in convincing researchers of the need for a more explicit and rigorous approach to diagnosis generally and the era of operationalized diagnostic methods began.

OPERATIONAL DEFINITIONS

The concept of operational definitions actually arose not from psychiatry or psychology but from physics, when Bridgman (1927), a physicist finding his branch of the subject in a state of conceptual turmoil, suggested the introduction of a new way of defining scientific concepts. He proposed that "an operational definition of a scientific term S, is a stipulation to the effect that S is to apply to all and only those cases for which performance of the test operation T, yields the specific outcome O." In other words, Bridgman proposed that to define S the researcher needs to set up a series of experiments for which the outcome is predicted. If the predicted outcome is observed for the complete set of experiments, then the definition of S is fulfilled. The philosopher, Hempel (1961) took this further. He suggested that Bridgman's concept could be introduced to psychiatry to overcome diagnostic difficulties with the modification that "the diagnosis S should be applied to all of those and only those manifesting the characteristic of satisfying the criterion O, subject to the proviso that O should be *objective* and *inter-subjectively* [*emphasis added*] certifiable and not something experienced intuitively or empathically by the examiner."

Essentially Hempel was suggesting that a focus on reliable and rigorously defined symptoms would allow them to be elicited in a way that was in effect a series of experiments, the outcomes of which could be tested. In addition, Hempel proposed that graded traits be converted to present/absent dichotomies by asking the question "Does the subject exhibit this much of X," where X is a symptom or item of psychopathology. We have pointed out elsewhere (Farmer et al. 2002) that the German psychopathologist Kurt Schneider, although he did not use the term *operational definition* and, as far as we know, was unaware of Bridgman's work, proposed a definition of schizophrenia in 1939 (translated into English in 1959) that was effectively an operational one (Schneider 1939/1959). Schneider proposed that schizophrenia could be diagnosed with confidence if there was "absence of coarse brain disease (a demonstrable brain lesion or metabolic disturbance)" and one or more "first rank" symptoms, these being a list of 10 symptoms that Schneider (1939/ 1959) judged from clinical experience to be of first-rank importance and that many subsequent studies (e.g., Brockington et al. 1978; McGuffin et al. 1984) have shown to be highly reliable.

The first operational criteria to be published de novo were the St. Louis criteria (Feighner et al. 1972). Although these criteria provide definitions of schizophrenia and affective disorder that are recognizably operational in structure as defined by Hempel, Feighner et al. neither cited Hempel's writing nor used the term *operational*. Indeed the practical attractions of these criteria for researchers proved to be more influential than any amount of theorizing about diagnostic processes, and their publication led to various other sets of operational criteria being proposed, culminating in the criteria set out in DSM-III (American Psychiatric Association 1980).

Although the introduction of DSM-III was a landmark in the history of psychiatric diagnosis, it must be remembered that operational definitions of disorder are attended by difficulties as well as by the obvious strength of improved reliability. We have discussed these in greater detail elsewhere (Farmer et al. 2002), but perhaps the most obvious difficulty is that DSM-III, and its successors DSM-III-R (American Psychiatric Association 1987), DSM-IV (American Psychiatric Association 1994), and DSM-IV-TR, are "official" sets of criteria that are expected to be used in the clinic as well as in research. However, although it is straightforward and desirable in research to adopt an algorithmic approach aided by standardized interviews and/or symptom checklists, it is not usually feasible or desirable to do so in clinical practice. Therefore, we strongly suspect that although clinicians in the United States and elsewhere would say that they apply DSM-IV-TR in their daily practice, there is often an element of self-deception in asserting this, because many of the criteria for common disorders are so complex that they are not easily adhered to in a way that is meticulous or precise. The other question mark hanging over DSM-IV-TR definitions of disorder is of course whether they are valid.

THE VALIDITY CONUNDRUM

In a classic and much quoted paper, Robins and Guze (1970) described a set of paths to establishing validity. These began with clinical studies to establish face validity and follow-up and outcome studies to establish stability of diagnostic categories and examine usefulness in predicting outcome. The next task was to establish whether the disorder "bred true" and ran in families. Last, Robins and Guze predicted that laboratory tests would eventually become useful in what were seen at the time as "functional" disorders and that these would be incorporated in an ultimately objective and valid classification. Given that our intent in this chapter is to discuss phenotypic problems in psychiatry, we focus largely on phenotype–genotype issues and therefore confine ourselves primarily to family genetic studies, using schizophrenia and affective disorders as our main examples.

Family and Genetic Studies of Schizophrenia

Fairly soon after operational definitions became commonplace in psychiatric research, papers began to appear (e.g., Abrams and Taylor 1983) suggesting that schizophrenia was no longer familial once "strict" definitions of the disorder were applied within family studies. Other authors protested that this was allowing the tail to wag the dog, because familiality was one of the best established epidemiological features of schizophrenia and thus a definition that did not support familiality must in itself be faulty and invalid. In fact, it subsequently turned out that failure to find familiality was probably a result of the methods that were applied, which lacked both sensitivity and power, and subsequent studies showed that operationally defined schizophrenia was indeed familial. Similarly, when operational definitions were applied to the Maudsley twin series previously studied by Gottesman and Shields (1972), a variety of definitions of schizophrenia, including the Feighner et al. (1972) criteria and DSM-III, proved to be associated with a high heritability of around 80% (Farmer et al. 1987; McGuffin et al. 1984). These criteria had also shown high reliability with kappa coefficients in the range of 0.75–0.85. However, that high reliability does not necessarily equate with validity (if we assume that a valid definition of schizophrenia should have heritability) is illustrated by Schneider's first-rank symptoms. In this reassessment of the Maudsley series, Schneider's (1939/1959) criteria were the most reliable of all, giving perfect agreement between raters and a kappa coefficient of 1.0. Despite this reliability, Schneider's first-rank symptoms defined a form of schizophrenia with 0 heritability.

If we continue with the same theme of examining the heritability of the definition of a disorder as a possible indicator of validity by turning to major depressive disorder, an interesting pattern emerges from twin study results. Kendler et al. (1992) carried out an important series of studies using their Virginia Twin Registry. Focusing initially on women, they applied a variety of diagnostic criteria, including those in DSM-III-R, to a large population-based sample that included 742 complete twin pairs. The estimated lifetime prevalence of depression varied, according to the definition applied, from 12% to 33%. The heritability of the disorder ranged from 21% to 45%, with no evidence of shared (or familial) environmental effects. Taking a somewhat different approach, McGuffin et al. (1996) studied a series of twins via probands who had been treated for depression at the Bethlem Royal and Maudsley Hospitals, London, and who were listed on the Maudsley Twin Register; 177 probands fulfilled DSM-IV criteria for at least one treated episode of major depression. McGuffin et al. (2003a), using an indirect method based on Camberwell case registry data (Camberwell is the old London borough in which the Maudsley Hospital is situated), calculated a lifetime morbid risk of around 8%. The heritability of major depression was estimated at 75%, and as in Kendler's twin study, there was no evidence of other than nonshared environmental effects.

At first sight it may seem odd that two different studies using ostensibly closely similar criteria should produce lifetime estimates that differ so markedly and heritabilities that differ by a factor of 2 or more. However, at least part of the differences must be attributed to the methods that were employed. It is perhaps not surprising that a study based on a treated sample of depressed twins should produce a lower estimate of the occurrence of depression in the population, because it is widely accepted that a proportion of depression goes unrecognized and untreated, and a population-based study will inevitably uncover a substantial number of such cases. The higher heritability in the clinically based sample (McGuffin et al. 1996) may also reflect the possibility that twins ascertained through clinics are more severally ill than those sampled in the community.

An indication that more severe depressive disorder is associated with higher heritability comes from a third twin series in which the registry was based on former U.S. military personnel from the Vietnam War era (Lyons et al. 1998). The size of the heritability estimates here was closer to those from the Virginia series than to those from the Maudsley series, but this in turn could reflect the likelihood that a sample of ex-military personnel will tend to be generally biased in the direction of better health.

Another factor that may vitiate the validity of the definition of a disorder is failure to remember symptoms. It is reasonable to assume that depression of sufficient severity to warrant treatment would be more memorable than less severe depression that was not treated. Rice et al. (1992) examined the stability of diagnosis in families ascertained through a depressed proband. Relatives were interviewed at two time points 6 years apart. Indicators of stability of lifetime diagnosis were examined—that is, the authors explored the factors predicting receiving a lifetime diagnosis of major depression at first interview and continuing to fulfill diagnostic criteria at second interview. Only 74% of those diagnosed with lifetime-ever depression at the initial interview still met criteria at the second interview. It was found that treatment and severity/number of symptoms significantly affected diagnostic stability. Ninety-six percent of treated cases with eight or more symptoms fell into the stable category. Kendler et al. (1993) found an even larger degree of diagnostic instability, or rather unreliability, in the Virginia female twins. The agreement on a lifetime diagnosis of depression based on interview and a self-completed questionnaire was modest ($\kappa = 0.34$). The authors derived an "index of caseness" based on the number of depressive symptoms, treatment seeking, number of episodes, and degree of impairment. They found that the higher the index of caseness, the better the reliability. They also found that the estimated heritability of lifetime major depression was greater for more restrictive definitions. The finding of multiple episodes being associated with higher heritability is a consistent result in other twin (Lyons et al. 1998; McGuffin et al. 1996) and family (Sullivan et al. 2000) studies. Kendler et al. (1993) then incorporated error of measurement into a structural equation model, including both occasions of measurement. The estimated heritability of the liability to depression increased substantially to approximately 70%. More than half of what was estimated as environmental effects, when lifetime major depression was analyzed on the basis of one assessment, was found to reflect measurement error when two assessments were used.

Therefore, in summary, there appears to be general agreement between recent twin study findings from clinic-based and population-based studies. Definitions of depressive disorder that are based on or incorporate treated disorder, more severe definitions, and definitions that include recurrence are associated with higher heritability estimates. More than one point of assessment can reduce reliability and increase heritability. The heritability estimates of major depression under these circumstances tend to converge on 70% rather than the often quoted figures of 30%–40% (Sullivan et al. 2000).

Of course, we set out in this section to discuss validity and cited Robin's and Guze's seminal article to justify exploring the extent to which the definition of a disorder affords high heritability. It could be argued that genes are only part of the etiological mix in the major psychiatric disorders, and we could just as well validate a definition according to whether it is highly associated with some specified environmental risk factors or set of factors. Where defining a disorder according to the "most genetic" definition unarguably comes into its own is when we are setting out with a specific task in mind: to locate and identify the genes involved in liability to a disorder. Here we begin to consider not just the validity but the utility of the definition of a phenotype.

Utility: The Extent to Which Diagnoses Are Useful

There are many other ways in which the utility of a diagnosis may be judged, including the extent to which it predicts course, outcome, treatment response, and so on. However, here we consider what is meant by *utility* within the context of neurobiological and specifically genetic etiology.

From all that we have discussed so far, there is an implication that, for the purposes of studies aimed at gene finding, restrictive definitions of disorder are likely to have the greatest utility. This would fit well with the current view, in studies of complex genetic traits that can be measured on a continuum, that one can achieve the greatest efficiency by concentrating on the extreme ends of distributions (Jawaid et al. 2002). The recent genetic studies on depression give a reasonably clear picture of what is meant by "restrictive": depression that is severe, recurrent, and associated with seeking treatment. With other disorders, in particular schizophrenia, the pattern is less clear cut.

This difficulty can be illustrated by comparing two studies that took a polydiagnostic approach to diagnosis—that is, they used not just one but several different diagnostic systems and applied them to the same group of patients. One of these was the original Maudsley Twin Series used by Gottesman and Shields (1972) to explore the genetics of schizophrenia. The other was a consecutive series of patients with a primary diagnosis of psychosis admitted to the psychiatric unit of King's College Hospital in London, a general teaching hospital that is just across the street from the Maudsley (Farmer et al. 1992).

Farmer et al. (1992) compared the results from these studies in an attempt to examine the relationship between different operational diagnostic criteria for schizophrenia. The data that they inspected consisted

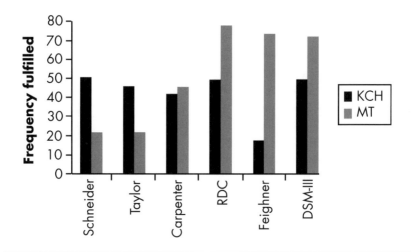

FIGURE 5–1.   Operational criteria for schizophrenia: frequencies in King's College Hospital (KCH) and Maudsley Twin (MT) Series.
RDC=Research Diagnostic Criteria.

of the frequency of operational definitions fulfilled by 60 index cases from a twin series and 144 consecutive admissions to King's College Hospital with a broad diagnosis of psychotic illness. The results are summarized in Figure 5–1. As shown in the figure, the relationship between the different criteria of schizophrenia is complicated and appears to be variable for different data sets. For the King's College series, the majority of subjects were considered to have schizophrenia on the basis of having one or more first-rank symptoms using the Schneider (1939/1959) criteria, whereas in the Maudsley series far fewer subjects fulfilled this definition. With the exception of the Research Diagnostic Criteria (Spitzer et al. 1978), which provided the broadest definition of schizophrenia in both samples, there was almost a reversal of the order of the frequencies of the different criteria fulfilled in each data set. Thus, the King's College series was mainly positive for the Schneider (1939/1959) definition, the criteria of Taylor and Abrams (1978), and the criteria of Carpenter et al. (1973). However, in the Maudsley twin series, the Research Diagnostic Criteria, DSM-III criteria, and the Feighner et al. (1972) criteria were the most commonly fulfilled.

These differences cannot be explained purely on the basis of rater differences, because two of three raters were the same in both studies. On the other hand, one of the differences was that the King's College series was selected on the basis of a broadly defined psychotic illness, whereas the Maudsley series was selected by specifically concentrating on schizophrenia. Nevertheless, this situation would not account for the low frequency of schizophrenia as defined by criteria of Schneider (1939/1959) used in the Maudsley series. Farmer et al. (1992) therefore suggested that the differences derived from two sources: first, the way in which the diagnostic information was collected and recorded, and second, from intrinsic differences in the clinical composition of the two series. In the Maudsley Twin Series the information was collected in a standard way according to a research protocol (Gottesman and Shields 1972) but without using a structured interview, and the principal researchers did not have a particularly "Schneider-oriented" view of psychopathology. By contrast, the King's College series was studied by a Schneider-oriented group of researchers using the Present State Examination, which, as noted earlier, tends to place important weight upon positive Schneiderian symptoms.

The difference in selection of each series was that the Maudsley series twins were ascertained via a hospital twin register that accumulated cases over a period of almost 20 years. The King's College sample, by contrast, consisted of consecutive acute admissions, including a portion of first-episode cases. Therefore, it might be expected that the twin series would have a higher proportion of positives on those definitions of schizophrenia, such as DSM-III and Feighner et al. (1972) criteria, that require a longer period of illness or that specify that a diagnosis of schizophrenia can apply only if there is failure to return to a premorbid level of functioning. Such criteria would therefore be fulfilled by only a minority of subjects in the King's College series.

The authors concluded that, in light of these findings, one needs to question the view commonly held then (and still held today by some) that certain definitions of schizophrenia are intrinsically "narrow" and "strict," whereas others are "broad" and "liberal." In the two samples that were compared, quite different patterns occurred for all sets of criteria other than the Research Diagnostic Criteria, so that for the Maudsley Twin Series a definition of schizophrenia based on Schneider's (1939/1959) first-rank symptoms was narrow, whereas the DSM-III definition was broad. Just the opposite occurred in the King's College series, where the Schneider definition was fairly broad and the DSM-III definition was narrow. Thus, the results appear to be crucially dependent on the way in which the clinical information was collected and recorded and in the way that the sample was collected.

Comparisons Across Studies

Bearing in mind the dependence of research diagnoses on these vagaries the question arises as to whether it is really possible to obtain a consistent signal in genetic studies that overcomes background noise. Despite the unreliability of diagnosis in the era before operational criteria, twin studies at least seemed to give consistent results in schizophrenia. What of studies carried out in the era after operational criteria? Five studies were reviewed and re-analyzed by Cardno and Gottesman (2000), and the results are summarized in Table 5–1. Essentially there is a high degree of agreement across the one Japanese and four European studies pointing to a very substantial genetic contribution, with a heritability in excess of 80%.

Does such consistency translate to studies designed to actually locate and identify genes? Until comparatively recently, the answer would have been no. Combining data from linkage studies creates additional problems over and above purely diagnostic ones. Such studies use different markers for their genome scans and different methods of analysis. Ingenious methods have been devised to overcome these difficulties. Badner and Gershon (2002) adapted a method originally proposed by Fisher (1932), whereas Levinson et al. (2003) divided the genome into segments, or "bins," and used a ranking method to assess the degree of support across studies for linkage within each segment. The two methods yielded overlapping but somewhat different results. The study of Badner and Gershon (2002) strongly supported the existence of susceptibility genes on chromosomes 8p, 13q and 22q, whereas that of Levinson et al. (2003) and Lewis et al. (2003) favored chromosomes 5q, 3p, 11q, 6p, 1q, 22q, 8p, 20q, and 14p. Thus, the 8p and 22q regions were supported by both meta-analyses, but eight other regions were supported by only one.

Nevertheless, despite the fact that there remain ambiguities surrounding linkage findings in schizophrenia, several groups have been sufficiently emboldened to embark on detailed searches within putative linkage regions. Their efforts led to the publication of a flurry of papers between 2002 and 2003 implicating several positional candidate genes in schizophrenia. Essentially, a *positional candidate* is a gene within a region of the genome identified by linkage studies that could plausibly be involved in the pathogenesis of the disorder, and there is now consistent evidence implicating *NRG-1*, a neuregulin gene in the linkage region on chromosome 8p, and the dysbindin gene, which is located in the linkage region of chromosome 6p, as well as highly suggestive evidence favor-

TABLE 5–1. Recent twin studies of schizophrenia

Authors	Country	Ascertainment	Diagnostic criteria	Monozygotic concordance	Dizygotic concordance	Heritability, %
Kläning (1996)	Denmark	Population register	ICD-10	7/16 (44%)	2/19 (11%)	83
Cannon et al. (1998)	Finland	Population register	ICD-8/DSM-III-R	40/87 (46%)	18/195 (9%)	
Franzek and Beckmann (1998)	Germany	Hospital admissions	DSM-III-R	20/31 (65%)	7/25 (28%)	
Cardno et al. (1999)	United Kingdom	Hospital register	DSM-III-R	20/47 (43%)	0/50 (0%)	84
			ICD-10	21/50 (42%)	1/58 (2%)	83
Tsujita et al. (1998)	Japan	Hospital admissions	DSM-III-R	11/22 (50%)	1/7 (14%)	
Combined			DSM-III-R	57/114 (50%)	4/97 (4.1%)	88
			ICD-10	28/66 (42.4%)	3/77 (3.9%)	83

Source. Data from Cardno and Gottesman 2000.

ing a role for *G72/DAAO* on 13q, *COMT* on 22q, and *RGS-4* on chromosome 1q (see reviews by McGuffin et al. 2003b; O'Donovan et al. 2003).

In summary, despite their imperfections, modern phenotypic definitions of disorders such as schizophrenia allow good enough agreement across studies to be useful in obtaining some general consensus on heritability estimates and even, most recently, in actually being able to identify genes. Some questions remain regarding the boundaries around disorders, the overlap between disorders, and the question of whether we are dealing with discrete categories or with dimensions.

COMORBIDITY, SYMPTOM CLUSTERS, AND DIMENSIONS

The recent advance in identifying linkage regions and positional candidate genes in schizophrenia has, for some onlookers, been marred by the emerging findings that at least some genomic regions, such as chromosomes 13q and 22q, appear to contain susceptibility genes for both schizophrenia and bipolar disorder (Badner and Gershon 2002). Indeed, a chromosome 13q candidate gene, *G72*, has been found to be associated with bipolar disorder. Inevitably this leads to the question of whether the classic Kraepelinian concept of two major psychoses is, after all, correct or whether there is either just one disorder, unitary psychosis, or what Crow (1990) has referred to as a continuum of psychosis, with schizophrenia at one end, bipolar disorder at the other, and mixed forms in between. A twin analysis using the Maudsley series suggested that neither of these hypotheses is correct. Cardno et al. (2002) analyzed their data in applying the diagnoses of schizophrenia, schizoaffective disorder, and bipolar disorder in a nonhierarchical fashion so that it was possible for a twin subject to have zero, one, two, or all three diagnoses. They then applied a trivariate structural equation modeling approach. The broad principles of this approach are shown in Figure 5–2. Essentially, the authors found that there are specific genetic effects on both schizophrenia and bipolar disorder but not on schizoaffective disorder. There were also genetic effects that were common to all three disorders. All three disorders also appeared to be influenced by disorder-specific nonfamily environments. These results would therefore predict that there will be some genes/linkage regions that are shared between bipolar disorder and schizophrenia and some that are specific to the two major disorders. Thus far, the molecular genetic data seem to be bearing out this prediction.

The Maudsley Twin Series has also been recently used to examine the relationship between bipolar disorder and unipolar depression (McGuf-

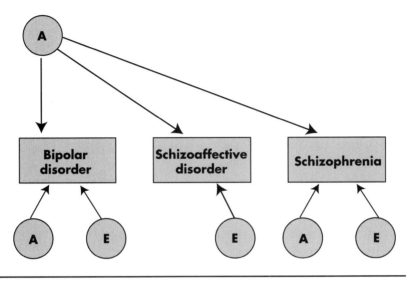

FIGURE 5–2. Path diagram showing that additive genetic effects (A) contribute to a shared liability to develop schizophrenia, schizoaffective disorder, and bipolar disorder.

There are specific nonfamily environmental effects (E) on all three syndromes but specific additive genetic effects only for schizophrenia and bipolar disorder.

Source. Data from Cardno et al. 2002.

fin et al. 2003a). A model in which bipolar disorder is simply a more severe, "more genetic" form of unipolar disorder could be rejected. The most satisfactory model was one in which there was a substantial overlap between the genes that confer liability to depression and mania, but most of the genetic contribution to a manic syndrome was specific to that syndrome. This again has implications for gene-finding studies. For example, many linkage studies of bipolar disorder classify both unipolar and bipolar relatives of bipolar probands as affected. The Maudsley Twin Series results suggest that some genes will only tend to be shared between pairs of relatives when both relatives have experienced mania.

It should be said that all such structural equation modeling depends on the basic assumption of a liability to disorder that only manifests as the disease when a certain threshold is exceeded (Falconer 1965; Reich et al. 1972). Therefore, we are conceptualizing these conditions as both categorical and dimensional. This brings us back to the issue of how best to define unipolar depression—broadly as in community-based studies or narrowly as in clinic-based research. This question is impossible to answer unless there exists some clear-cut boundary between disorder and "normal" symptoms of depression, which does not appear to be the case. Instead, there appears to be a shading from normality into abnormality, and because depression is usually an episodic disorder, this shading is compounded by state as well as trait effects. Indeed, the whole question of the extent to which vulnerability to depression—or its obverse, resilience in the face of adversity—is tied up with personality traits is a topic of much current interest (Farmer et al. 2003) and leads to the even thornier issue of the relationship between what we now call Axis I disorders and disorders of personality.

The question of whether psychopathology is better measured and described dimensionally rather than categorically is nowhere more pressing than in the case of personality disorder. This is so because dimensional approaches are now universally accepted as the better and more useful way of describing normal personality, whereas a categorical approach remains the dominant and officially sanctioned way of describing personality disorder, despite widespread dissatisfaction with the current classification schemes. Not long after the introduction of DSM-III, Frances (1982) defended the categorical method in personality diagnosis, pointing out that there are many things in nature that are better viewed categorically even if this does not capture the total reality or reliably distinguish subtle shades of difference. Color variation is a good example of a phenomenon that we know results from continuous variation within the visible spectrum, but, nevertheless, referring to colors as distinct-named categories is "quite handy when one wants to buy a suit or describe a sunset." On the other hand, for some tasks involving light waves, such as a study of refraction, a dimensional system is more precise and contains more information. The argument then is that for everyday purposes, categories win out because they are "simple and convenient abstractions of what is essential."

CONCLUSION

The search for the solution to the phenotype problem has come a long way but has not gone away or even reached the stage when it can be downgraded to a puzzle. Explicit or operational diagnostic criteria coupled with standardized interviews have dramatically improved reliability, even if operational criteria pose some new problems for clinical practice. Modern definitions of psychiatric phenotypes are valid in as much as they describe categories of high heritability. Quantitative genetic studies have led to studies that are now successfully exploring the molecular genetic etiology of common psychiatric disorders. However, our current classification does not define disorders that are mutually exclusive either phenotypically or etiologically. For example, both the statistical and the molecular genetic evidence suggests that some genes are associated with an increased risk of both schizophrenia and bipolar disorder. Part of our difficulty arises from the clinical necessity of applying categories to phenomena whose underlying structure is almost certainly dimensional. The ultimate solution to the phenotype problem will need to include some rational way of accommodating this necessity.

REFERENCES

Abrams R, Taylor MA: The genetics of schizophrenia: a reassessment using modern criteria. Am J Psychiatry 140:171–175, 1983

American Psychiatric Association: Diagnostic and Statistical Manual: Mental Disorders. Washington, DC, American Psychiatric Association, 1952

American Psychiatric Association: Diagnostic and Statistical Manual of Mental Disorders, 3rd Edition. Washington, DC, American Psychiatric Association, 1980

American Psychiatric Association: Diagnostic and Statistical Manual of Mental Disorders, 3rd Edition, Revised. Washington, DC, American Psychiatric Association, 1987

American Psychiatric Association: Diagnostic and Statistical Manual of Mental Disorders, 4th Edition. Washington, DC, American Psychiatric Association, 1994

American Psychiatric Association: Diagnostic and Statistical Manual of Mental Disorders, 4th Edition, Text Revision. Washington, DC, American Psychiatric Association, 2000

Badner JA, Gershon ES: Meta-analysis of whole-genome linkage scans of bipolar disorder and schizophrenia. Mol Psychiatry 7:405–411, 2002

Beck AT, Ward CH, Mendelson M, et al: Reliability of psychiatric diagnoses, 2: a study of the consistency of clinical judgments and ratings. Am J Psychiatry 119:351–357, 1962

Bridgman PW: The Logic of Modern Physics. New York, Macmillan, 1927

Brockington JF, Kendell RE, Leff JP: Definitions of schizophrenia: concordance and prediction of outcome. Psychol Med 8:387–398, 1978

Cannon TD, Kaprio J, Lonnqvist J, et al: The genetic epidemiology of schizophrenia in a Finnish twin cohort: a population-based modeling study. Arch Gen Psychiatry 55:67–74, 1998

Cannon TD, Marshall EJ, Coid B, et al: Heritability estimates for psychotic disorders: the Maudsley twin psychosis series. Arch Gen Psychiatry 56:162–168, 1999

Cardno AG, Gottesman II: Twin studies of schizophrenia: from bow-and-arrow concordances to star wars Mx and functional genomics. Am J Med Genet 97: 12–17, 2000

Cardno AG, Rijsdijk FV, Sham PC, et al: A twin study of genetic relationships between psychotic symptoms. Am J Psychiatry 159:539–545, 2002

Carpenter WT, Strauss JS, Bartko JJ: Flexible system for the diagnosis of schizophrenia: a report from the WHO pilot study of schizophrenia. Science 182: 1275–1278, 1973

Cooper JE, Kendell RE, Gurland BJ, et al: Psychiatric Diagnosis in New York and London. London, Oxford University Press, 1972

Crow TJ: The continuum of psychosis and its genetic origins: the sixty-fifth Maudsley lecture. Br J Psychiatry 156:788–797, 1990

Edmonds D, Eidinow J: Wittgenstein's Poker. New York, Harper Collins, 2001

Falconer DS: The inheritance of liability to certain diseases, estimated from the incidence among relatives. Ann Hum Genet 29:51–76, 1965

Farmer AE, McGuffin P, Spitznagel EL: A cluster analytic approach to schizophrenia. Psychiatry Res 8:1–12, 1983

Farmer AE, Katz R, McGuffin P, et al: A comparison of the composite diagnostic interview (CIDI) and the present state examination (PSE). Arch Gen Psychiatry 44:1064–1068, 1987

Farmer AE, Wessely S, Castle D, et al: Methodological issues in using polydiagnostic approach to define psychotic illness. Br J Psychiatry 161:824–830, 1992

Farmer A, McGuffin P, Williams J: Measuring Psychopathology. Oxford, England, Oxford University Press, 2002

Farmer A, Mahmood A, Redman K, et al: A sib-pair study of the Temperament and Character Inventory scales in major depression. Arch Gen Psychiatry 60:490–496, 2003

Feighner JP, Robins E, Guze SB, et al: Diagnostic criteria for use in psychiatric research. Arch Gen Psychiatry 26:57–67, 1972

Fisher RA: Statistical methods for Research Workers. London, Oliver & Boyd, 1932

Frances A: Categorical and dimensional systems of personality diagnosis: a comparison. Compr Psychiatry 23:516–527, 1982

Franzek E, Beckmann H: Different genetic background of schizophrenia spectrum psychoses: a twin study. Am J Psychiatry 155:76–83, 1998

Gottesman II, Shields J: Schizophrenia: A Think Study Vantage Point. New York, Academic Press, 1972

Hempel CG: Introduction to problems of taxonomy, in Field Studies in the Mental Disorders. Edited by Zubin J. New York, Grune & Stratton, 1961, pp 3–22

Jawaid A, Bader JS, Purcell S, et al: Optimal selection strategies for QTL mapping using pooled DNA samples. Eur J Hum Genet 10:125–132, 2002

Kendler KS, Neale MC, Kessler RC, et al: A population-based twin study of major depression in women: the impact of varying definitions of illness. Arch Gen Psychiatry 49:257–266, 1992

Kendler KS, Neale MC, Kessler RC, et al: The lifetime history of major depression in women: reliability of diagnosis and heritability. Arch Gen Psychiatry 50:863–870, 1993

Klaning U, Mortensen PB, Kyvik KO: Increased occurrence of schizophrenia and other psychiatric illnesses among twins. Br J Psychiatry 168:688–692, 1996

Kramer M: Some problems for international research suggested by observations as differences in first admission rates to mental hospitals of England and Wales and of the United States, in Proceedings of the Third World Congress of Psychiatry, Vol. 3. Montreal, Quebec, Canada, University of Toronto Press, 1961, pp 153–160

Levinson DF, Levinson MD, Segurado R, et al: Genome scan meta-analysis of schizophrenia and bipolar disorder, part I: methods and power analysis. Am J Hum Genet 73:17–33, 2003

Lewis CM, Levinson DF, Wise LH, et al: Genome scan meta-analysis of schizophrenia and bipolar disorder, part II: schizophrenia. Am J Hum Genet 73: 34–48, 2003

Lyons MJ, Eisen SA, Goldberg J, et al: A registry-based twin study of depression in men. Arch Gen Psychiatry 55:468–472, 1998

McGuffin P, Farmer AE, Gottesman II, et al: Twin concordance for operationally defined schizophrenia: confirmation of familiality and heritability. Arch Gen Psychiatry 41:541–545, 1984

McGuffin P, Katz R, Watkins S, et al: A hospital-based twin register of the heritability of DSM-IV unipolar depression. Arch Gen Psychiatry 53:129–136, 1996

McGuffin P, Rijsdijk F, Andrew M, et al: Heritability of bipolar affective disorder and the genetic relationship to unipolar depression. Arch Gen Psychiatry 60:497–502, 2003a

McGuffin P, Tandon K, Corsico A: Linkage and association studies of schizophrenia. Curr Psychiatry Rep 5:121–127, 2003b

O'Donovan MC, Williams NM, Owen MJ: Recent advances in the genetics of schizophrenia. Hum Mol Genet 12:R125–R33, 2003

Reich T, James JW, Morris CA: The use of multiple thresholds in determining the mode of transmission of semi-continuous traits. Ann Hum Genet 36:163–184, 1972

Rice JP, Rochberg N, Endicott J, et al: Stability of psychiatric diagnoses: an application to the affective disorders. Arch Gen Psychiatry 49:824–830, 1992

Robins E, Guze SB: Establishment of diagnostic validity in psychiatric illness: its application to schizophrenia. Am J Psychiatry 126:983–987, 1970

Schneider K: Clinical Psychopathology (1939). Translated by Hamilton M. New York, Grune & Stratton, 1959

Spitzer RL, Endicott JR: Schedule of Affective Disorders and Schizophrenia, 3rd Edition. New York, Biometrics Research, 1978

Sullivan PF, Neale MC, Kendler KS: Genetic epidemiology of major depression: review and meta-analysis. Am J Psychiatry 157:1552–1562, 2000

Taylor MA, Abrams R: The prevalence of schizophrenia: a reassessment using modern diagnostic criteria. Am J Psychiatry 135:945–948, 1978

Tsujita T, Niikawa N, Yamashita H, et al: Genomic discordance between monozygotic twins discordant for schizophrenia. Am J Psychiatry 155:422–424, 1998

Wing JK, Cooper JE, Sartorius N: Measurement and Classification of Psychiatric Symptoms. Cambridge, England, Cambridge University Press, 1974

World Health Organization: Report on International Pilot Study of Schizophrenia, Vol 1. Geneva, World Health Organization, 1973

CHAPTER 6

Advancing
From Reliability
to Validity

The Challenge for the DSM-V/ICD-11 Revisions

Darrel A. Regier, M.D., M.P.H.

William E. Narrow, M.D., M.P.H.

Donald S. Rae, M.S.

Maritza Rubio-Stipec, D.Sc.

Speaking before the American Psychopathological Association in 2000, Robert Kendell (2002) listed five criteria for improving the taxonomy of mental disorders. He noted that two criteria—making the diagnostic system more comprehensive and making it more complex as disorders are dissected and subdivided into smaller homogeneous groups—may seemingly conflict with a third aim of making it easier to use. A fourth criterion was to devise a more objective means of establishing disorder thresholds than reliance on "clinical significance" criteria. Finally, he pointed out the need for improvements in either reliability or validity. Kendell also contributed significantly to a chapter by Rounsaville et al.

(2002) in *A Research Agenda for DSM-V* (Kupfer et al. 2002) that identified how some of the validity criteria established by Robins and Guze
(1970) could lead to contradictory conclusions about the nature of disorders—for example, genetic aggregation criteria could lead to different
conclusions about the nature of underlying pathology than might clinical course and delimited syndrome criteria. Adhering to the model, one
could be left with a conflicting hierarchy of validity criteria for identifying the most significant measure of diagnostic validity. In another seminal paper published shortly before Kendell's untimely death, Kendell
and Jablensky (2003) presented a stellar discussion on "distinguishing
between the validity and utility of psychiatric diagnosis." That paper
afforded a useful starting point for considering how to advance from reliability to validity in future revisions of DSM and ICD classifications.

Because the first author's (D.A.R.) research has been in the field of
epidemiology, we focus in this chapter on developments in epidemiology that have tested the validity of existing criteria and can continue to
contribute to the evidence base for future revisions. However, the American Psychiatric Association has an interest in drawing on the full range
of research, from neuroscience to cross-cultural studies, for revisions of
the classification systems. For an appreciation of this breadth of interest,
the reader is referred to the monograph (Kupfer et al. 2002) that compiled
"white papers" from six workgroups charged to explore how to expand
the scientific base for psychiatric classification. We conclude this chapter with a preview of next steps toward this goal for future iterations of
DSM and ICD classifications—specifically, DSM-V and ICD-11.

DSM AND ICD: A BRIEF HISTORY OF DEVELOPMENT

Over the second half of the twentieth century, the field progressed from
concepts of validity focused on presumed etiology of mental disorders
as "reactions" either to unconscious conflicts or to known environmental
stressors (in DSM-I [American Psychiatric Association 1952] and DSM-II
[American Psychiatric Association 1968]) to an atheoretical emphasis
(as far as etiology is concerned) on reliability that focuses on identifying
syndromes with explicit criteria that can be observed and replicated
across settings. The criteria in DSM-III (American Psychiatric Association 1980) were intended to be hypotheses that were subject to empirical
testing. Upon their introduction, these criteria were incorporated into the
Diagnostic Interview Schedule (DIS; Robins et al. 1981), which was used
with more than 20,000 Epidemiologic Catchment Area (ECA) subjects
during the next 4 years (Regier et al. 1984). Findings of high comorbidity

between so-called primary disorders higher on a diagnostic hierarchy such as schizophrenia and other disorders specifically listed in the exclusion criteria such as panic disorder led to dropping diagnostic hierarchies from DSM-III-R (American Psychiatric Association 1987), whereas emerging clinical evidence led to expanding criteria for certain disorders such as social phobia. The failure of DSM-III criteria to specifically define individuals with only one disorder should, in retrospect, have served as an alert that a strict neo-Kraeplinian categorical approach to mental disorder diagnoses, advocated by Robins and Guze (1970), Spitzer et al. (1978), and others, could have some serious problems.

Faith in a strict categorical approach persisted, however, and the DSM-III-R criteria were also incorporated into the Composite International Diagnostic Interview (CIDI; Robins et al. 1988), an international version of the DIS, sponsored by the World Health Organization (WHO), that was modified by Kessler as a University of Michigan version (Wittchen and Kessler 1994) for the National Comorbidity Survey (NCS; Kessler 1994; Kessler et al. 1994). A combination of the broader criteria and the use of single-item stem questions as screeners resulted in even higher levels of individual disorders and of comorbid disorders.

DIAGNOSIS, CLINICAL SIGNIFICANCE, AND NEED FOR TREATMENT

Much has been made of the high rates of disorders found in the NCS, the ECA, and even the few community studies that used the Schedule for Affective Disorders and Schizophrenia–Lifetime Version for assessing Research Diagnostic Criteria disorders in the community (Weissman et al. 1978). Some commentators have noted that the high rates were seen as a problem only because of the stigma associated with mental disorders and that comparably high rates for any physical disorder would not raise eyebrows. However, the most troubling fact about these high rates was that in the few studies in which measures of functional impairment such as the Global Assessment Scale (GAS; Endicott et al. 1976; later defined as the Global Assessment of Function [GAF] scale contained in Axis V of DSM-III-R) were used, as many as 50% of respondents scored above 70, which is the cutoff for mild impairment (Regier et al. 1985). This finding raised questions about the "missing criteria" that were not contained in DSM-III or DSM-III-R and that differentiated those who met criteria and felt a need to seek mental health services from those who met full criteria but experienced no such need to seek care. Because it is difficult to conceive of any definition of mental disorder that does not involve some level of dysfunction, the authors of DSM-IV (American Psychiatric Association 1994) felt that the way to deal with this issue was to add a "clinical significance" criterion that required significant distress or impairment for all disorders.

Many who participated in the development of the DIS and, subsequently, the ECA study (Regier et al. 1984) were confident that the new descriptive criteria of DSM-III would be sufficient to screen out those with true disorders from those with no psychopathology. However, in order to collect diagnostic information from a community population with lay interviewers, it was necessary to develop a fully structured interview that would replicate clinical decision processes that psychiatrists or other mental health professionals use in evaluating the significance of symptoms. As noted in the introduction to DSM-IV, this "inherently difficult" effort helps to establish a disorder threshold and requires clinical judgment processes.

Lee Robins took the lead in developing the probe-flowchart that cross-examined the subject on each symptom with the aim of separating the trivial from the significant. Although some critics have contended that the probe-flowchart simply confused service use with disorders, that was not the intent of the questions, and there is ample evidence to show that that was also not the effect. The intent was to replicate a clinician's evaluation of symptoms, which includes a determination of their severity by seeing if they rose sufficiently for a patient to tell a professional of some kind about the symptoms, to take any kind of over-the-counter or prescription medicine for the symptoms, or to feel that the symptoms interfered to a noteworthy extent with their life activities. Because many of the people who mentioned their symptoms to a professional, perhaps in the course of social service or medical visits, never specifically sought mental health services for such symptoms in any setting, one can argue that the probe-flowchart provided the most minimal assessment of clinical significance and did not use service utilization as a validator of disorder (Wakefield and Spitzer 2002a).

When the NCS rates emerged at even higher levels for a single interview than were found for the ECA, a group at the National Institute of Mental Health in the mid-1990s began a detailed analysis of the potential causes for discrepancies. One readily apparent potential cause was that the University of Michigan version of the CIDI used a slightly different probe-flowchart. Beyond this variation, differences between population groups, instrument construction, and diagnostic criteria (DSM-III vs. DSM-III-R) were examined, with subsequent publication of the results (Regier et al. 1998). When the differences in available measures of clinical significance or severity were analyzed, it became apparent that all members of the ECA team had completely forgotten that the "clinical significance" data collected from the interview sections for some *syndromes*, as opposed to probe-flowchart assessments of their component *symptoms*, had not been used in the scoring of disorder rates in either the ECA or the NCS (Narrow et al. 2002; Regier and Narrow 2002). The reanalysis afforded an opportunity to evaluate the impact of using these additional criteria on prevalence rates and correlates of the defined mental disorders. Upon the authors' presentation of these data at the American Psychopathological Association meeting in 2000, Wakefield and Spitzer (2002a, 2002b) issued a strong critique contending that clinical significance criteria were misguided. They called for additional criteria that would make it possible to add greater levels of specificity to the disorder definitions to include contextual information and implied that an extension of Axis IV of DSM might serve as a vehicle for such criteria. Implicit in their critique was an intent to maintain the purity of their somewhat "reified" diagnoses, which needed to be separated from orthogonal concepts of disability and distress.

In retrospect, it is remarkable that investigators involved in developing the scoring algorithms for the DIS failed to use information similar to that in the probe-flowchart that qualified the clinical significance of symptoms for qualifying the clinical significance of diagnostic syndromes. As Kendell and Jablensky (2003) observed, investigators fell into the trap of reifying tentative definitions of mental disorders as reflecting true underlying psychopathology if the requisite symptoms were simply present in the right combination and of sufficient duration, without paying adequate attention to their intensity or severity when grouped together for diagnostic syndromes. Remarkably, even clinicians who were asked to reevaluate community subjects as part of the validation phase of the DIS found almost equally high rates of disorders even though there were variable kappa levels describing the match between those subjects identified by both methods (Anthony et al. 1985).

In this context, the trenchant critique of Kendell and Jablensky about the implicit "disease entity" assumptions of Robins and Guze is relevant:

> The weakness of the validity criteria of both Robins and Guze and Kendler was that those criteria implicitly assumed that psychiatric disorders are discrete entities and that the role of validity criteria is to determine whether a putative disorder, such as "good-prognosis schizophrenia" or paranoia, is a valid entity in its own right or a mild form or variant of some

other entity. The possibility that disorders might merge into one another with no natural boundary in between—what Sneath called a "point of rarity," but what is better regarded as a zone of rarity—was simply not considered. (Kendell and Jablensky 2003, p. 5)

In fairness, it should be noted that the Robins and Guze (1970) criteria were written at a time when there was still a strong belief among many, if not most, American psychiatrists that psychoanalysis offered the only comprehensive theory of mental disorder etiology and treatment, in which all psychiatric disorders were on a continuum from normality to neurosis to psychosis, to be explained primarily by the previously mentioned unconscious conflicts or severe environmental stresses producing war neuroses or early forms of posttraumatic stress disorder. The St. Louis group, known as the neo-Kraeplinians, presented a medical model of the day in which discrete diagnostic entities such as bipolar disorder and schizophrenia were expected to have only a few genes explaining their biological vulnerabilities. Likewise, there were few studies designed to demonstrate natural boundaries between syndromes defined according to the Feighner et al. (1972) criteria or between such syndromes and normality.

The foregoing discussion suggests that two principal critiques of DSM-IV (and its update, DSM-IV-TR; American Psychiatric Association 2000) can be drawn from more than 30 years of research: 1) that prevalence rates for mental and behavioral disorders are too high to develop a clinically meaningful and, from a public health perspective, logistically feasible response to them and 2) that existing validity criteria for mental disorders are limited and contradictory.

ADDING DIMENSIONALITY TO A CATEGORICAL CLASSIFICATION SYSTEM

These criticisms, however, should be viewed in the larger context of general medicine. Recent research has identified diseases throughout medicine for which vulnerability is polygenetic, onset or occurrence is dependent on various environmental exposures, and expressed disease processes appear to extend in a continuous manner from normal to pathological. Examples of these include hypertension, type 2 diabetes, hypercholesterolemia, and one of particular interest to the first author, Ehlers-Danlos syndrome, which entails abnormalities of connective tissue. This syndrome subsumes at least nine genetic subtypes—involving, for example, skin hyperelasticity, hypermobility of joints, and tissue fragility—that can extend to serious vascular and other organ complications (Germain 2002). In families with these disorders, there is often no correlation between genotype and phenotype because of the varied molecular mechanisms that have been observed with different mutations in each family. If mood disorders eventually prove to have even the same modest number of genetic subtypes, one could attempt for an indefinite period of time to identify precise syndrome boundaries between subtle genetic mutations without ever defining a "valid syndrome" in the Robins and Guze framework. In such cases, one can only approximate the syndromes with manifestational criteria until genetic subtypes are identified along with minor mutations due to spontaneous variations or environmental exposures that can lead to a "valid" understanding of the syndrome.

Again, the conclusion reached by Kendell and Jablensky (2003) is relevant:

> discrete disease entities and dimensions of continuous variation are not mutually exclusive means of conceptualizing psychiatric disorders: both are compatible with a threshold model of disease and may account for different or even overlapping segments of psychiatric morbidity. Second, the surface phenomena of psychiatric illness (i.e., the clustering of symptoms, signs, course, and outcome) provide no secure basis for deciding whether a diagnostic class or rubric is valid, in the sense of delineating a specific, necessary, and sufficient biological mechanism. (pp. 6–7)

Conceptually, categorical approaches include the following: the criteria describe separate underlying pathophysiological entities that have a normal distribution from mild to severe, and concepts of disability and distress are orthogonal to underlying diagnostic entities and ideally should be measured separately from diagnosis. Wakefield and Spitzer (2002a) developed a Venn diagram illustrating the relationships between disorder, distress, and disability. In contrast, a dimensional approach views illnesses as reflecting a combination of symptoms, on a continuum with normality, and requiring cutpoints derived from statistical associations with clinical course outcomes.

In reality, psychiatric nosology has been using a combination of categorical and dimensional approaches already in a number of areas including clinical treatment, clinical trials research, the *Global Burden of Disease* assessments (Murray and Lopez 2000), and—in attempting to address an issue of particular interest to the American Psychopathological Association—the generation of accurate definitions of incidence, remission, recovery, and relapse (Frank et al. 1991). The benefit of having epidemiological studies that have incorporated these criteria is that they provide a useful evidence base for evaluating the consequences of various alternative approaches to diagnosis. For example, changes in unipolar major depression and dysthymia prevalence rates are fairly striking when the syndrome-specific "clinical significance" information is actually used as intended in the scoring of the ECA and NCS studies. The overall rates of disorders dropped substantially and are still not equivalent to current concepts of "medical necessity" or "need for treatment" (Narrow et al. 2002).

The correlates of employment status, disability compensation, suicidal ideation and attempts, and the percentage of individuals using services, are indicative of a higher level of "predictive validity."

DIAGNOSIS AS A PREDICTOR OF NEED FOR SERVICES

To those who feel that the syndrome-specific questions confuse service use with diagnosis, it is interesting to note that these are the same questions that were used to evaluate the clinical significance of individual symptoms in the DIS and CIDI. Arguably, if they are not useful for syndrome definition, they are similarly not useful for the entire symptom foundation of the DIS and CIDI instruments. On an empirical level, one can see that positive responses are not isomorphic with service use; Narrow et al. (2002) found that almost 50% of respondents with positive diagnoses failed to use mental health services in the year of diagnosis. Building on this experience, the authors have identified several strategies for using epidemiological data to assist in DSM revisions.

Powerful as the epidemiological data may be to record the consequences of discrepancies in criteria for prevalence rates and correlations with risk factors and service use, they are essentially most useful in identifying "zones of rarity" between useful categorical syndromes or in setting thresholds for continuous measures. As Kendell and Jablensky (2003) noted,

> If the *defining characteristic* of the category is a syndrome, this syndrome must be demonstrated to be an entity, separated from neighboring syndromes and normality by a zone of rarity. Alternatively, if the category's defining characteristics are more fundamental—that is, if the category is defined by a physiological, anatomical, histological, chromosomal, or molecular abnormality—clear, qualitative differences must exist between these defining characteristics and those of other conditions with a similar syndrome. (p. 8)

In Kendell and Jablensky's framework, "the crucial issue in determining validity is not understanding of etiology but rather the existence of clear boundaries or qualitative differences at the level of the defining characteristic" (p. 8). Epidemiological data gathered from many countries around the world, generated by both the DIS and CIDI instruments, can now be mined to determine if zones of rarity between different definitions of disorders can be found in these large population groups. In some such data sets, additional genetic samples have been taken that may eventually be used to identify more fundamental characteristics of specific mental disorders.

CONCLUSION

With the support and collaboration of the National Institutes of Health, the WHO, and the World Psychiatric Association, the American Psychiatric Association hopes to enlist the assistance of the entire range of research investigators to assess both categorical and dimensional aspects of psychopathology. Contributions to our understanding of valid disorder concepts and criteria can emerge from multiple research disciplines and fields of inquiry that have been addressing mental disorders since the early 1990s, when both DSM-IV and ICD-10 were released. Undoubtedly, this work will lead to new paradigms for describing the boundaries and continuities between disorders. One can hope that the increased precision that is possible with improved diagnoses will be linked to an increased potential for both prevention and treatment interventions that directly address pathological deviations in brain physiology due to both genetic predisposition and toxic environmental exposure.

REFERENCES

American Psychiatric Association: Diagnostic and Statistical Manual: Mental Disorders. Washington, DC, American Psychiatric Association, 1952

American Psychiatric Association: Diagnostic and Statistical Manual of Mental Disorders, 2nd Edition. Washington, DC, American Psychiatric Association, 1968

American Psychiatric Association: Diagnostic and Statistical Manual of Mental Disorders, 3rd Edition. Washington, DC, American Psychiatric Association, 1980

American Psychiatric Association: Diagnostic and Statistical Manual of Mental Disorders, 3rd Edition, Revised. Washington, DC, American Psychiatric Association, 1987

American Psychiatric Association: Diagnostic and Statistical Manual of Mental Disorders, 4th Edition. Washington, DC, American Psychiatric Association, 1994

American Psychiatric Association: Diagnostic and Statistical Manual of Mental Disorders, 4th Edition, Text Revision. Washington, DC, American Psychiatric Association, 2000

Anthony JC, Folstein M, Romanoski AJ, et al: Comparison of lay Diagnostic Interview Schedule and a standardized psychiatric diagnosis. Arch Gen Psychiatry 42:667–675, 1985

Endicott J, Spitzer RL, Fleiss JL, et al: The Global Assessment Scale: a procedure for measuring overall severity of psychiatric disturbance. Arch Gen Psychiatry 33:766–771, 1976

Feighner JP, Robins E, Guze SB, et al: Diagnostic criteria for use in psychiatric research. Arch Gen Psychiatry 26:57–63, 1972

Frank E, Prien RF, Jarrett RB, et al: Conceptualization and rationale for consensus definition of terms in major depressive disorder. Arch Gen Psychiatry 48:851–855, 1991

Germain DP: Clinical and genetic features of vascular Ehlers-Danlos syndrome. Ann Vasc Surg 16:391–397, 2002

Kendell R: Five criteria for an improved taxonomy of mental disorders, in Psychopathology in the 21st Century: DSM-V and Beyond. Edited by Helzer JE, Hudziak JJ. Washington, DC, American Psychiatric Association, 2002, pp 3–19

Kendell R, Jablensky A: Distinguishing between the validity and utility of psychiatric diagnoses. Am J Psychiatry 160:4–12, 2003

Kessler RC: The National Comorbidity Survey: preliminary results and future directions. Int J Methods Psychiatr Res 4:114.1–114.13, 1994

Kessler RC, McGonagle KA, Zhao S, et al: Lifetime and 12-month prevalence of DSM-III-R psychiatric disorders in the United States: results from the National Comorbidity Survey. Arch Gen Psychiatry 15:8–19, 1994

Kupfer DJ, First MB, Regier DA (eds): A Research Agenda for the DSM-V. Washington, DC, American Psychiatric Association, 2002

Murray CJL, Lopez AD (eds): The Global Burden of Disease. Cambridge, MA, Harvard University Press, 2000

Narrow WE, Rae DS, Robins LN, et al: Revised prevalence estimates of mental disorders in the United States: using a clinical significance criterion to reconcile 2 surveys' estimates. Arch Gen Psychiatry 59:115–123, 2002

Regier DA, Narrow WE: Defining clinically significant psychopathology with epidemiological data, in Psychopathology in the 21st Century: DSM-V and Beyond. Edited by Helzer JE, Hudziak JJ. Washington, DC, American Psychiatric Association, 2002, pp 19–30

Regier DA, Myers JK, Kramer M, et al: The NIMH Epidemiologic Catchment Area program: historical context, major objectives, and study population characteristics. Arch Gen Psychiatry 41:934–941, 1984

Regier DA, Burke JD, Manderscheid RW, et al: The chronically mentally ill in primary care. Psychol Med 15:265–273, 1985

Regier DA, Kaelber CT, Rae DS, et al: Limitations of diagnostic criteria and assessment instruments for mental disorders: implications for research and policy. Arch Gen Psychiatry 55:109–115, 1998

Robins E, Guze SB: Establishment of diagnostic validity in psychiatric illness: its application to schizophrenia. Am J Psychiatry 126:983–987, 1970

Robins LN, Helzer JE, Croughan J, et al: National Institute of Mental Health Diagnostic Interview Schedule: its history, characteristics, and validity. Arch Gen Psychiatry 38:381–389, 1981

Robins LN, Wing J, Wittchen HU, et al: The Composite International Diagnostic Interview: an epidemiologic instrument suitable for use in conjunction with different diagnostic systems in different cultures. Arch Gen Psychiatry 45: 1069–1077, 1988

Rounsaville BJ, Alcaron RD, Andrews G, et al: Basic nomenclature issues for DSM-V, in A Research Agenda for DSM-V. Edited by Kupfer DJ, First MB, Regier DA. Washington, DC, American Psychiatric Association, 2002, pp 1–29

Spitzer RL, Endicott J, Robins E: Research diagnostic criteria: rationale and reliability. Arch Gen Psychiatry 35:773–782, 1978

Wakefield JC, Spitzer RL: Lowered estimates: but of what? (commentary). Arch Gen Psychiatry 59:129–130, 2002a

Wakefield JC, Spitzer RL: Why requiring clinical significance does not solve epidemiology's and DSM's validity problem: response to Regier and Narrow, in Psychopathology in the 21st Century: DSM-V and Beyond. Edited by Helzer JE, Hudziak JJ. Washington, DC, American Psychiatric Association, 2002b, pp 31–40

Weissman MM, Myers JK, Harding PS: Psychiatric disorders in a U.S. urban community, 1975–1976. Am J Psychiatry 135:459–462, 1978

Wittchen HU, Kessler RC: Modifications of the CIDI in the National Comorbidity Survey: the development of the UM-CIDI. January 1994. Available at: http://www.hcp.med.harvard.edu/ncs/um-cidi.pdf. Accessed March 28, 2003.

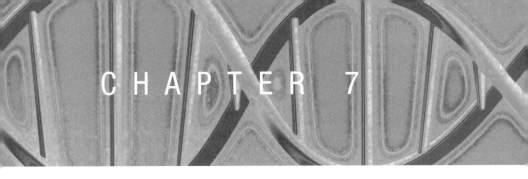

CHAPTER 7

Prospects for Prevention of Mental Disorders in the Era of Genomic Medicine

Linda B. Cottler, Ph.D.

THE HUMAN GENOME PROJECT

Two months after the 93rd annual meeting of the American Psychopathological Association (APPA), all of the main goals established by a National Academy of Sciences panel to sequence the human DNA code were achieved. The project, called the Human Genome Project (HGP; U.S. Department of Energy Human Genome Project 2003), was a partnership between the U.S. government, international agencies, and private businesses. Centers in the United Kingdom, France, Germany, Japan, and China worked with scientists in the United States to sequence the 3 billion "letters" of human DNA. The National Human Genome Research Institute at the National Institutes of Health, which funded U.S. scientists to complete the project, is coordinating the application of this work to the public's health. According to Dr. Francis Collins, the current Director of the Institute, their work is just beginning (Collins 2003) as it turns its focus to the application of genomics to three major areas: biology, health, and society (Collins et al. 2003).

In the genomics-to-biology phase, all of the functions of each gene will be identified, and the genetic networks and protein pathways will be established. One of the challenges of this focus will be to understand the "heritable variation in the human genome" (Collins et al. 2003); this will require the development of a catalog of all variants in the sequencing of genetic material to understand who acquires illness X or Y. Studies are investigating the most common form of variation—single nucleotide polymorphisms (SNPs). Because SNPs are inherited in blocks or haplotypes, mapping these through the International HAPMAP Project will enable investigators to find common patterns of base pair sequences among persons with illness X or Y.

In the genomics-to-health phase, investigators are working to understand how genetic factors affect health and illness as well as the individual response to pharmaceutical interventions and how those same factors interact with nongenetic (or environmental) factors. It is this focus that could revolutionize the classification of illness as well as subsequently determine who is at risk for certain therapies. As stated by Collins et al. (2003):

> The time is right for a focused effort to understand, and potentially reclassify, all human illnesses on the basis of detailed molecular characterization. Systematic analyses of somatic mutations, epigenetic modifications, gene expression, protein expression and protein modification should allow the definition of a new molecular taxonomy of illness, which would replace our present, largely empirical classification schemes and advance both disease prevention and treatment.

Focusing on the genomics-to-society phase requires investigators to deal with the ethical, legal, and social implications of the HGP. This endeavor could help uncover the association between genomics and race and ethnicity as well as individual or group "identity." Although this area of pursuit should allow for a reduction in health disparities, it could simultaneously increase them as well. Employers who gain access to information about one's genetic makeup could alter hiring practices or restrict one's job classification—a high likelihood for persons with mental disorders and other stigmatizing high risk behaviors and lower socioeconomic status.

With the completion of the original goals of the HGP, the sequencing of the entire human genome, optimists believe it is a matter of time before people will be able to learn about their individual risks for many illnesses such as cancer, diabetes, Alzheimer's disease, and others. It is even hypothesized that by 2020, the diagnosis and treatment of mental disorders will be "transformed" (Collins 2003). Medical records could contain a person's complete genome, including SNPs, which could potentially help determine the response to certain drugs as well as individual vulnerability to the illness. However informed we are of our genotype or specific SNPs, this information will be neither sufficient nor necessary to predict our development of symptoms or progression to illness. Health and illness are determined not only by genetic and environmental factors but also by chance, which is random and cannot be predicted.

In this chapter, I review issues relevant to prevention of mental disorders and discuss some of the major challenges to the field of public health psychiatry as it begins to grapple with the discovery of genetic information and its potential usefulness for the early prevention of mental disorders. Although the field is in its infancy, its magnitude as well as its importance to psychiatry was marked in the history of the APPA at our 95th annual meeting in 2005, which was devoted exclusively to the topic of early prevention of mental disorders.

POTENTIAL FOR PREVENTION OF MENTAL DISORDERS IN THE ERA OF THE GENOME

Tackling the issue of prevention of mental disorders, with or without information on the genome, is daunting. There are numerous disorders in DSM-IV-TR (American Psychiatric Association 2000) and numerous categories of illnesses including addictions, internalizing and externalizing disorders, impulse-control disorders, stress disorders, mood disorders, and many others. The notion that each has a unique, underlying genetic basis has been challenged (Kendler 1996). Also, because of the widespread condition of comorbidity, pure cases are rare. Prevention messages become complicated by varying patterns of symptom onset, duration, and diagnostic exclusions. Additionally, disorders such as posttraumatic stress disorder, substance abuse and dependence, and pathological gambling are conditional on exposure, and investigators have found unique predictors for exposure and subsequent development of these illnesses. This situation warrants separate prevention messages to be crafted for the exposure and for the consequences of exposure.

CHALLENGES FOR PREVENTION IN GENERAL

Although the HGP is transforming disease prevention and treatment, the widest gap between the sequencing of genes and the immediate utility of such information exists for psychiatry. Merikangas and Avenevoli (2000) described several phenomena that can be used to explain why the

gap is so wide—that is, why the genotype may not predict the phenotype and vice versa. These include *penetrance*, or the probability of a
gene to express itself; *variable expressivity*, the degree to which individuals with the gene express various components of it; *gene–environment
interaction*, which is the expression of the genotype in the presence of
certain nongenetic factors; *pleiotropy*, or the ability of one gene to cause
many different traits; and *genetic heterogeneity*, in which different genes
express themselves identically.

These phenomena explain why we do not know with certainty who
will develop a mental illness and thus who could benefit from targeted
prevention efforts. The need to prevent mental illnesses is irrefutable,
however. With lifetime prevalence rates around 50% and rates of current
mental disorders in the range of 15%–25%, they are among the most
common conditions on the planet (Kessler 2002). Surveys from multiple
international sites also show that besides being among the most common, they are among the most disabling, most chronic (with ages at onset occurring earlier than most every other chronic disorder), and least
confined (most mental disorders occur along with at least one other) (Kessler 2002). Prevention of mental illnesses would have a great impact on
society.

The manner in which these illnesses should best be prevented, as
well as the timing of prevention efforts, has yet to be determined. Kessler (2002) and others have noted the need for interventions for certain
disorders as early as childhood or adolescence, because it is unknown
whether childhood disorders are premorbid or precursor conditions for
disorders later in life or represent unique manifestations of disorders on
their own. Prevention science is defined by appropriately matching prevention strategies with disease stage. The types of efforts are presented
in the next section.

PREVENTION STRATEGIES

Although the matching of effort depends on many factors, including the
progression of the illness and the type of condition, the goal of the effort
is to increase and enhance *protective factors* that can lower risk; reverse
risk factors (elements that, when present, are associated with a greater
likelihood of a behavior than when not present); and eliminate illness
altogether. In 1994, the Institute of Medicine proposed a change in the labeling of these strategies from terms we have become accustomed to—
primary, *secondary*, and *tertiary*—to *universal*, *selective*, and *indicated*.

Universal Strategies

Universal strategies, also known as community-based and primary prevention strategies, address a community—whether at the national, local, school, or neighborhood level—to prevent or delay the initiation of a behavior or set of symptoms. Examples of such strategies include the Drug and Alcohol Resistance Education (DARE) school program, the National Rifle Association's Eddie Eagle gun safety program for elementary school–age children, vaccinations to prevent infectious diseases, prenatal education, and public service announcements. Universal, community-based programs address issues among all individuals, regardless of risk level, assuming that all members of a population share a similar general risk for a disorder, even though the risk varies from person to person. As expressed by Geoffrey Rose (1992) in his influential work, "A large number of people exposed to a small risk may generate many more cases than a small number of people exposed to a high risk" (p. 24), since "even a small shift at the peak of a risk curve can have sizeable population effects" (p. 24). Additionally, an intervention for coronary heart disease could have profound benefits to the population for other illnesses, such as stroke and high blood pressure, that are related to coronary heart disease, a primary cause of death for persons age 55 years and older.

In a recent review of the literature from the previous 20 years, Merzel and D'Afflitti (2003) emphasized that many community-based, universal prevention programs intervening in the areas of cardiovascular disease, smoking, cancer, substance abuse, and immunizations have not met with much success. Reasons for a lack of effect range from methodological issues (such as low statistical power and design and sampling issues, including poor response rates), secular trends (changes in societal attitudes), modest effect sizes, and limitations in the interventions (short durations, insufficient tailoring, and low-level penetration) to limitations in the theoretical underpinnings of the prevention message chosen. Additionally, the universal message may be too diluted to affect people or may cause listeners to tune out if no personal gain is perceived from the message. Merzel and D'Afflitti also discussed lessons for all fields of medicine to be learned from HIV prevention, including reliance on self-report rather than exclusive reliance on medical records; an emphasis on changing social norms using peers; use of formative research, including ethnographic and qualitative methods; the severity of the illness; and the homogeneity of the targeted communities.

Selective Strategies

Selective strategies, which are similar to secondary prevention strategies, are targeted at subgroups of a population with characteristics that place them at higher risk than the general population for an illness. Examples of such groups might include children of divorced or depressed parents (to prevent externalizing disorders or depressed mood and its later progression to depression) and children of crack/cocaine users or parents with alcoholism (to prevent substance use, abuse, and dependence). These strategies might also be used in geographic areas where there is high drug availability to target specific groups of kids about more detailed drug prevention messages. Selective strategies target groups at risk by virtue of their risk, even though persons within the groups may exhibit varying levels of risk. An individual's risk is not the target in this type of prevention effort.

Indicated Strategies

Indicated strategies, similar to tertiary prevention efforts, are designed to prevent more serious complications among persons showing some signs of illness to reduce the duration and lessen the severity of the symptoms. Examples might include prevention efforts or early therapy among youth who test positive for drugs but who have not received a diagnosis of substance use disorder; use of medication to prevent osteoporosis in women; needle exchange programs among injection drug users; and antipsychotic use among schizophrenic patients to achieve better outcomes.

Indicated and selective strategies, so-called high-risk strategies, are thought to be more appropriate than universal strategies among persons specifically exhibiting some risk factors because they target the persons who need the message, which presumably increases the saliency of the message. Furthermore, these strategies may be more cost-effective, and if there are side effects, they will be experienced only among those who could benefit from the therapy.

However, because science cannot predict with certainty which persons are likely to develop an illness, it also cannot predict who among those at "higher risk" could benefit from these strategies. This situation speaks to a need to direct prevention efforts at persons at lowest risk, where most of the cases of illness occur. Rose (1992) described the drawback of limiting prevention to only those who are at high risk, using data from the U.K. Heart Disease Prevention Project (Heller et al. 1984). In this trial, 15% of the men were found to have some risk factors without early signs of disease. At the 5-year follow-up, only 7% of those men were found to have had a myocardial infarction (MI). More importantly, 93% had been found to be well at follow-up. The 7% MI rate represented only one-third of all of the MIs that occurred in the group as a whole. If prevention strategies had been limited to only those men labeled at elevated risk with early symptoms, only 2% of the population would have been affected. Although 22% of the men in this group had an MI over the 5 years of follow-up, 78% did not. Furthermore, only 12% of all MIs occurred in the men in this group; fully 88% of the MIs occurred in a lower-risk group. These data demonstrate that "what is best for the selected individuals is worst for the community."

In fact, high-risk prevention strategies may actually do more harm than good, as evidenced by findings from Dishion and colleagues at the University of Oregon Child and Family Center. Youths 11–14 years of age at high risk for drug abuse and exhibiting some signs of aggression and delinquency were grouped together for a 12-week program designed to reduce problem behavior. Those who were grouped with their peers were found to exhibit significantly worse behaviors, as measured by their average scores on the Child Behavior Checklist at 12 weeks and at the 1-, 2-, and 3-year follow-ups, compared with those who either were given materials to study on their own or received no intervention at all (Dishion et al. 1999; Poulin et al. 2001).

CHALLENGES FOR PREVENTION STRATEGIES IN PUBLIC HEALTH PSYCHIATRY

The challenges facing public health psychiatry are unique relative to other branches of medicine specifically due to the phenomena discussed earlier (Merikangas and Avenevoli 2000). Additionally, there are other issues unique to psychiatry that must be accounted for in prevention strategies, including case ascertainment, case definition, assessment of the disorder, and a potpourri of risk and protective factors.

Case Ascertainment

Berkson's bias (Berkson 1946)—the finding that there is a stronger association between two disorders among people admitted to a hospital or to treatment compared with people from the general population—explains why some prevention messages may be less effective for persons with less perceived need for treatment or intervention. Many etiological findings have originated from clinical samples and thus are unrepresentative, biased, and uninformative for choosing prevention strategies.

Case Definition

In DSM-I (American Psychiatric Association 1952) there were only 130 pages and 35,000 words, and DSM-II (American Psychiatric Association 1968) had only 135 pages. Thus, pure cases were common. Beginning with DSM-III (American Psychiatric Association 1980), however, and continuing through DSM-IV-TR, there are now close to 1,000 pages and hundreds of disorders allowing for multiple diagnostic labels. The validity of so many disorders with few or no tangible biological markers has been questioned. Creative approaches for addressing validity were first proposed by Robins and Guze (1970) in their landmark paper, in which they identified five phases in establishing validity: describing the psychopathology, laboratory findings, delimitation from other disorders, stability of disorders over time, and a family history of illness similar to that in the index subject.

Diagnostic Assessment

Within the limits of this chapter, the controversial subject of diagnostic assessments cannot be properly discussed. However, no discussion of case definition or assessments would be complete without acknowledging the historical significance of the first generation of modern diagnostic studies, the Epidemiologic Catchment Area study, and the second-generation study, the National Comorbidity Survey (Kessler 2002). These studies developed and fine-tuned mechanisms for obtaining diagnostic information from subjects themselves, using nonclinician interviewers, that could be used to generate a better understanding of the behaviors people, in or out of treatment, experience. Thus, for the first time, it became possible to gain insight into which persons might be at increased risk for the development of a psychiatric disorder, to discover the threshold age for illness (outside of treatment samples), to determine the prodromal period for a disorder, and to comprehend the meaning of co-occurring psychopathologies.

Risk and Protective Factors

Finally, the potpourri of risk and protective factors specific to our branch of medicine is beginning to be more fully elucidated by epidemiological studies under way, suggesting more appropriate designs and choices for prevention messages. However, as Kraemer et al. (2001) pointed out, the collection of data on risk factors and how they mediate or moderate an effect is tricky. The authors stated that interventions designed around factors that are fixed, that cannot be changed, are "a waste of time." Also, when an intervention addresses only one causal link in a larger chain, little policy significance can result. Additionally, the collection of risk factor data without a temporal ordering of those factors and the symptoms they purportedly "cause" cannot establish directionality. Many studies have not included such questions because they are time consuming to administer, tricky to write, and difficult to assess; thus, it is impossible to determine groups or individuals with greater or lesser likelihood for benefiting from prevention messages. After decades of study, one thing is certain: psychiatric disorders are complex disorders attributed to many genes and environmental factors (Tsuang and Faraone 2000).

HIGH-RISK VERSUS UNIVERSAL PREVENTION: WHAT HAS BEEN TRIED, AND WHERE ARE WE HEADED?

Beyond the data presented to us by the HGP, the field will search for aspects of behavior that are modifiable—aspects that include environmental and nongenetic conditions. Some of these factors have already been identified for specific common disorders. We discuss the promise of high-risk versus universal prevention in the context of three disorders—schizophrenia, pathological gambling, and drug dependence. Although an exhaustive review of the progress made is beyond the scope of this chapter, the salient features of the endeavor are described to whet our appetite for a future volume.

Schizophrenia

High-risk strategies for the prevention of schizophrenia have been attempted for years, based on biological indicators. For example, schizophrenia has been associated with decreased gray matter and increased ventricular volume (Hulshoff Pol et al. 2001) even among patients who have never received antipsychotics, which have been known to cause similar structural changes. Other biological factors found among persons with schizophrenia are itemized in Jablensky's (2000) review of schizophrenia and include lower fertility rates, increased suicide rates, and higher than usual rates of substance dependence, physical illnesses, and organic brain disorders. "Gene profiling" in the areas of the brain that are affected could help identify high-risk persons susceptible to symptoms of schizophrenia later in life.

Although schizophrenia has been researched with various epidemiological approaches for more than 100 years (Jablensky 1995), it is only recently that investigators have suggested that this disorder could be prevented through universal strategies. Such a plan is not endorsed by everyone—some believe the only effective strategies that should be tried are those that are high risk, and then only among persons who have manifested precursor symptoms without the disorder (Mrazek and Haggerty 1994). Universal prevention could focus on the multitude of antecedents and risk factors possibly connected to schizophrenia, which include familial, environmental, social, and family factors. In the area of familial risk, the most powerful risk factor for schizophrenia, studies have found that the lifetime risk for developing this disorder increases 10-fold among first-degree relatives of persons with schizophrenia and nearly 50-fold if both parents have the disorder (Gottesman 1991). This would seem to argue for a high-risk strategy; however, as Mojtabai et al. (2003) pointed out, there is a low positive predictive value of family history as a risk factor. Specifically, 90% of first-degree relatives of probands with schizophrenia never develop the illness; false-negative cases occur at high rates, with two-thirds of persons with schizophrenia having no first-degree relative with the illness (Gottesman 1991). Thus, although familial factors are powerful, they have a smaller overall contribution to the total incidence of schizophrenia, compared with environmental factors. In fact, as stated by Murray and Castle (2000), if all cases among affected first-degree relatives could be eliminated, only one-tenth of the total number of cases would be prevented.

In terms of environmental factors, better prenatal care could help reduce obstetrical complications such as hypoxia, low birth weight, and premature births, which have been associated, albeit tenuously, with schizophrenia developed later in life (Geddes and Lawrie 1995). Seasonality, increased exposure to viruses, and in utero exposure to flu could also be weakly related to schizophrenia and preventable, although the strength of the association for each is low (Mednick et al. 1988). Finally, social and family factors affecting the likelihood for schizophrenia could be targets of universal interventions, especially among persons in an economically disadvantaged group, persons who are siblings of second-generation African-Caribbeans with schizophrenia (Hutchinson et al. 1996), and those living in urban areas and those who are not married (Jablensky 2000). One intriguing finding that warrants further study, and subsequent universal prevention efforts if found to be strong, is the association between cannabis use and schizophrenia, especially among users with other risk factors (Andreasson et al. 1987).

Although universal measures could be advantageous because of the obvious health benefits to a larger number of people for many different outcomes besides schizophrenia, they have not been initiated, even though the association between variables has been strong, biologically plausible, supported by a dose-response effect, and modifiable. These tenets are the same ones that have determined the strength of associations throughout the history of epidemiological research.

Perhaps the field is more comfortable with early intervention rather than universal intervention. Recent work has centered on the identification of prodromal states preceding the index episode of schizophrenia (Poulton et al. 2000). This type of work is predicated on the notion that a "reasonably accurate ability to predict who will develop schizophrenia is a necessary precondition for prevention trials" but is far from sufficient (Faraone et al. 2001, p. 10). According to Tsuang (personal communication 2003), a high-risk strategy should be attempted, beginning with early interventions first among young adults and then in younger cohorts until the age at onset for a syndrome of liability (schizotaxia) is found. Another approach will be to find specific endophenotypes (such as cognitive deficits or P50 abnormalities) to determine whether they lie along a single genetic dimension or multiple dimensions. Are we close to using biology or genetics for the prevention of schizophrenia? The answer is "no," but as the studies begin to define liability, we will be able to determine who to target for interventions. Doesn't this argue, then, for universal messages?

Pathological Gambling

An increasingly important public health problem is that of problem and pathological gambling. Pathological gambling is listed in DSM-IV-TR as an impulse-control disorder, although there are several competing etiological frameworks for the disorder, ranging from disorder of impulse control to mood disorder to obsessive-compulsive disorder to addictive disorder (Blanco et al. 2001; Potenza et al. 2003). In fact, the criteria mimic addictive disorders, with the disorder conditional on exposure and with craving, loss of control, withdrawal, and tolerance. Brain images of persons exposed to gambling cues show effects similar to drug cravings and compulsions (Moreyra et al. 2000; Potenza 2001). Perhaps as interesting as the case definition and biological effects is the involvement of the American Gaming Association in the issuance of universal messages to prevent problem gambling. Such involvement on the part of the casino industry is a deliberate attempt to thwart the bad image that the tobacco industry has earned. Prevention messages are ubiquitous at gambling venues and sponsored by the gaming industry; they include 1–800 BETS-OFF messages on slot cards, in bathrooms at casinos, on slot machines, on posters easily visible to patrons, and on lottery tickets. In fact, Missouri was the first state to initiate a Disassociated Persons List, which is a voluntary exclusion program to allow gamblers to ban themselves from entering a casino under penalty of arrest. (There are as of the time of this writing nearly 6,000 names on the list in Missouri.) Although the advertisement of the program is a universal prevention message, the list itself becomes a high-risk prevention strategy, although it has not yet been evaluated for its effectiveness.

There are familial, genetic, environmental, and biological components to pathological gambling. For example, as Eisen et al. (1998) have shown with a sample of about 3,500 male twin pairs, familial factors explained 62% of the variance in pathological gambling. They also found that about 50% of criteria, such as trying to cut down and gambling in larger amounts, was attributed to genetic influences. Winters and Rich (1999) found a dose-response gradient in that heritability was found for high-action gamblers compared with low-action gamblers. Environmental factors are also related to pathological gambling and are a source for risk. For example, in the past decade there has been a proliferation of casino venues and games, increasing the exposure rate of gambling among adults to nearly 90%, which is blamed on a potential increase in the incidence of problem gambling and ultimately, pathological gambling. High comorbidity with addictive disorders adds to the confusion about the classification of this disorder and the type of prevention message that would be most effective. Finally, in terms of biological issues, pathological gamblers have been found to exhibit a serotonergic deficit, and a noradrenergic dysfunction consistent with extraversion, compared with control subjects (Moreyra et al. 2000).

Perhaps the future will bring more universal messages, such as "Facing the Odds" (Harvard School Division on Addictions 2005), a basic primer for elementary school–age children that teaches statistics and odds as a primary prevention for the cognitive distortion that occurs with gambling. Such strategies are necessary, given that the rates of youth pathological gambling disorder are four times the rates seen in adults (Volberg 1994). However, until the nosology of the disorder is better understood, the genetic factors better elucidated, and the comorbidities sorted out between this and other illnesses, pathological gambling remains one in which a large number of people exposed to a small risk may generate many more cases than a small number exposed to a high risk. Thus, this behavior deserves continued community-wide messages at the youngest age possible.

Drug Dependence

Much has been written recently on prevention of substance abuse problems, and the field has reviewed the current state of research and tackled problems with design, feasibility, and evaluation with the public's health in mind (Merikangas and Clayton 2001). The implications of using family studies for prevention of substance use disorders were outlined (Merikangas and Avenevoli 2000) in the journal *Addictive Behaviors*, which followed on the heels of a special international conference on prevention. The series suggested numerous universal and high-risk strategies for prevention, and the reader is directed there for a concise yet thorough review of the literature ranging from the selection of models, to community prevention, school-based and family approaches, and policy-relevant approaches.

Several issues should be mentioned that are associated with universal prevention strategies for drug use, abuse, and dependence. First, increased availability of information to our teens may thwart our best intentions for prevention. All one needs to do is surf the web for "informational" sites regarding new trends in inhalants, party drugs, and flower seeds such as "morning glory" to see what our youth are learning about drug availability, consequences, and drug actions (see www.erowid.org). In our National Institute on Drug Abuse (NIDA)–funded study of the consequences of MDMA (3,4-methylenedioxymethamphetamine), one 24-year-old female user reported,

> I can use drugs professionally. I'm a professional drug user in the fact that I've used drugs since I was 16, and I've used quite a few. Even when I was 17 and 18, I felt that after I had initially gotten the gist of it that I knew what my boundaries were. I knew when and where to go to do it. I knew the effects that I was going to have so I would plan for what I was going to do.

Another user, also a 24-year-old female, said, "Just use 5HTP on Monday, and you'll restore your serotonin." These responses were given at the same time NIDA's Monitoring the Future study was declaring a slight reduction in prevalence of use of these drugs among twelfth graders and a concomitant increase in perceived risk. The question for NIDA remains: at what age should prevention messages be initiated? A meta-analysis found that teens may be more prone to risk-taking behaviors, such as drug use (and gambling and unprotected sexual behaviors), because brain development starts from the back of the brain to the front; frontal lobes are necessary for executive functioning, and that area of the brain matures later than other areas. Consequently, the teenage years may be the best and worst time to initiate prevention messages. What is necessary is science-based and repeated messages.

As discussed previously, fixed variables cannot be changed, and targeting them represents a waste of efforts (Kraemer et al. 2001); however, many risk factors exist that could be moderated, and those are the ones that deserve our attention. Examples include individual, family, school, and community factors. Family factors, which may offer our best hope, include history of drug use, family conflict, and lenient parental attitudes about using drugs. In a study we conducted in a local area high school, reported alcohol use was four times greater among students who perceived that their parents would let them drink (Cottler et al. 2001), compared with those who thought their parents would disapprove. Risk factors can be moderated by protective factors. These data were used in area-wide parent–teacher organization meetings to educate parents about staying in touch with other parents and monitoring their children's behavior more closely. They also bolstered the need for published phone books with indicators given for parents who would not sign a pledge stating that they would not allow or give alcohol to minors in their home.

Data from a six-state survey of sixth- to twelfth-grade students show that the prevalence of cannabis use increases as unmoderated risk factors increase (Hawkins et al. 2002). Prevention science postulates that drug use or alcohol use can be prevented or minimized if risk factors are reduced and protective factors increased. Hawkins' Communities That Care project plotted risk and protective factors in specific geographic locations to visually determine higher-risk and lower-risk communities to help prevention teams to more easily view, in three-dimensional format, which areas must be targeted for what and for whom. This was a unique use of "targeted" universal prevention messages.

AN EXCITING TIME FOR THE FUTURE: NEXT STEPS

This is an exciting time. It is a time when epidemiologists are needed more than ever to help elucidate the risk factors, the case definition, and many other conditions related to health and disease. The genome has been mapped, but that could be done in the confines of a laboratory, with computers and other equipment. The hardest part is yet to come— blending the sciences together in a meaningful way. This difficult assignment requires the human laboratory, where no two person's answers are the same, where extreme efforts are needed to achieve the expected high response rates (Cottler et al. 1996), where minority populations must be recruited and included, where ethics must never be overlooked in favor of information, and where quality control of data collection should be a necessary but not sufficient ongoing element of all epidemiological studies. Prevention in the era of the genome must also be culturally acceptable, yet globally transferable.

The next steps require us to also consider psychiatric enviromics (Anthony 2001) in the mix of genomics. This is the deliberate and systematic search for all modifiable nongenetic factors known (or unknown). As Anthony (2001) stated, this search could begin with an update of a catalog of every possible exposure variable with a manual on how to intervene at various points of the life span. It would also assess lifetime, comorbid conditions in order to understand biology, risk factors, and behaviors.

Epidemiologists who are fluent in neurobiology and neurobiologists who are fluent in epidemiology are needed. Epidemiological studies will be required to collect biological specimens to understand more fully the total picture of health and disease. Although public health professionals are more aware of risk factors than biological factors, a new framework for the field is in order—a framework initiated by Kandel (1998) that proposes that we become more knowledgeable about the structure and functioning of the brain in order to understand the interaction of social and biological determinants of behavior.

Blending prevention strategies with knowledge is proving to be a difficult task. As Merikangas and Risch (2003) noted recently, results from family and genetic studies have shown a peculiar finding—for smoking, spousal correlations and sibling correlations are equivalent, peer influences outweigh sibling histories, and there is a low parent–child concordance. The authors suggested that for smoking, research should focus more on social transmission—a malleable environmental risk factor for many disorders. They suggested that universal prevention messages will have more benefits than identifying the genes for individual smokers.

One suggestion is shown in Figure 7–1: if the risk factors, protective factors, genetic factors, and biological results are all unknown, it is in-

	Risk factors	Protective factors	Genetic results	Biological results
Universal	Unknown	Unknown	Unknown	Unknown
Selective	Probable	Probable	Probable	Probable
Indicated	Definite	Definite	Definite	Definite

FIGURE 7–1.   Prevention matrix.

cumbent on us to launch universal messages. If results of any of the factors are probable "causes" of the outcome, it is important that we launch a combination of universal and selective strategies. If we definitely understand which risk, protective, genetic, and biological markers are responsible for outcome X, it is our responsibility to launch a full-scale prevention effort that mixes universal, selective, and, most importantly, indicated strategies. Determining what research efforts should be planned should depend on the public health impact of the disease. As Rose (1992) noted so eloquently, a small reduction in risk for a large number of people could have much more impact on the public's health than a large reduction in risk for a small number of people.

REFERENCES

American Psychiatric Association: Diagnostic and Statistical Manual: Mental Disorders. Washington, DC, American Psychiatric Association, 1952
American Psychiatric Association: Diagnostic and Statistical Manual of Mental Disorders, 2nd Edition. Washington, DC, American Psychiatric Association, 1968
American Psychiatric Association: Diagnostic and Statistical Manual of Mental Disorders, 3rd Edition. Washington, DC, American Psychiatric Association, 1980

American Psychiatric Association: Diagnostic and Statistical Manual of Mental Disorders, 4th Edition, Text Revision. Washington, DC, American Psychiatric Association, 2000

Andreasson S, Allebeck P, Engstrom A, et al: Cannabis and schizophrenia: a longitudinal study of Swedish conscripts. Lancet 2:1483–1486, 1987

Anthony J: The promise of enviromics. Br J Psychiatry 40(suppl):S8–S11, 2001

Berkson J: Limitations of the application of fourfold table analysis to hospital data. Biometrics 2:47–53, 1946

Blanco C, Moreyra P, Nunes EV, et al: Pathological gambling: addiction or compulsion? Semin Clin Neuropsychiatry 6:167–176, 2001

Collins FS: The future of genomics. Testimony before the Subcommittee on Health, Committee on Energy and Commerce, United States House of Representatives, Washington, DC, May 22, 2003

Collins FS, Green ED, Guttmacher ED, et al: A vision for the future of genomics research. Nature 422:835–847, 2003

Cottler LB, Compton WM, Ben Abdallah A, et al: Achieving a 96.6% follow-up rate in a longitudinal study of drug abusers. Drug Alcohol Depend 41:209–217, 1996

Cottler LB, Ben Abdallah A, Compton W, et al: Association between attitudes and substance use among high school students. Presented at the 63rd annual meeting of the College on Problems of Drug Dependence. Scottsdale, AZ, June 2001

Dishion TJ, McCord J, Poulin F: When interventions harm: peer groups and problem behavior. Am Psychol 54:755–764, 1999

Eisen S, Lin N, Lyons MJ, et al: Familial influences on gambling behavior: an analysis of 3,359 twin pairs. Addiction 93:1375–1384, 1998

Faraone S, Green AI, Seidman LJ, et al: "Schizotaxia": clinical implications and new directions for research. Schizophr Bull 27:1–18, 2001

Geddes JR, Lawrie SM: Obstetric complications and schizophrenia: a meta-analysis. Br J Psychiatry 167:786–793, 1995

Gottesman I: Schizophrenia Genesis: the Origins of Madness. New York, WH Freeman, 1991

Harvard Medical School Division on Addictions: Facing the odds: the mathematics of gambling and other risks. Available at: http://www.divisiononaddictions.org/html/facingtheodds_form.htm. Accessed June 1, 2005.

Hawkins JD, Catalano RF, Arthur MW: Promoting science-based prevention in communities. Addict Behav 27:951–976, 2002

Heller RF, Chinn S, Tunstall-Pedoe IID, et al: How well can we predict coronary heart disease? Findings in the United Kingdom Heart Disease Prevention Project. BMJ 288:1409–1411, 1984

Hulshoff Pol HE, Schnack HG, Mandl RC, et al: Focal gray matter density changes in schizophrenia. Arch Gen Psychiatry 58:1118–1125, 2001

Hutchinson G, Takei N, Bhugra D, et al: Morbid risk of schizophrenia in first degree relatives of white and African-Caribbean patients with psychosis. Br J Psychiatry 169:776–780, 1996

Jablensky A: Schizophrenia: recent epidemiologic issues. Epidemiol Rev 17:10–20, 1995

Jablensky A: Epidemiology of schizophrenia, in New Oxford Textbook of Psychiatry. Edited by Gelder MG, Lopez-Ibor JJ, Andreason NC. Oxford, England, Oxford University Press, 2000, pp 585–598

Kandel ER: A new intellectual framework for psychiatry. Am J Psychiatry 155: 457–469, 1998

Kendler KS: Major depression and generalized anxiety disorder: same genes, (partly) different environments, revisited. Br J Psychiatry 168(suppl):68–75, 1996

Kessler R: Current issues in psychiatric epidemiology. Curr Opin Psychiatry 15: 181–186, 2002

Kraemer HC, Stice ES, Kazdin A, et al: How do risk factors work together? Mediators, moderators and independent, overlapping, and proxy risk factors. Am J Psychiatry 158:848–856, 2001

Mednick SA, Machon RA, Huttunen MO, et al: Adult schizophrenia following prenatal exposure to an influenza epidemic. Arch Gen Psychiatry 45:189–192, 1988

Merikangas K, Avenevoli S: Implications of genetic epidemiology for the prevention of substance use disorders. Addict Behav 25:807–820, 2000

Merikangas K, Clayton R: Introduction to the special issue of addictive behaviors. Addict Behav 25:805, 2001

Merikangas K, Risch N: Genomic priorities and public health. Science 302:599–601, 2003

Merzel C, D'Afflitti J: Reconsidering community-based health promotion: promise, performance, and potential. Am J Public Health 93:557–574, 2003

Mojtabai R, Malaspina D, Susser E: The concept of population prevention: application to schizophrenia. Schizophr Bull 29:791–801, 2003

Moreyra P, Ibáñez A, Saiz-Ruiz J, et al: Review of the phenomenology, etiology and treatment of pathological gambling. German Journal of Psychiatry 3:37–52, 2000

Mrazek PJ, Haggerty RJ (eds): Reducing Risk for Mental Disorders. Washington, DC, National Academy Press, 1994

Murray RM, Castle DJ: Genetic and environmental risk factors for schizophrenia, in New Oxford Textbook of Psychiatry. Edited by Gelder MG, Lopez-Ibor JJ, Andreason NC. Oxford, England, Oxford University Press, 2000, pp 599 605

Poulin F, Dishion TJ, Burraston B: Three-year iatrogenic effects associated with aggregating high-risk adolescents in cognitive-behavioral preventive interventions. Applied Development Science 5:214–224, 2001

Poulton R, Caspi A, Moffitt TE, et al: Children's self-reported psychotic symptoms and adult schizophreniform disorder: a 15-year longitudinal study. Arch Gen Psychiatry 57:1053–1058, 2000

Potenza MN: The neurobiology of pathological gambling. Semin Clin Neuropsychiatry 6:217–226, 2001

Potenza MN, Steinberg MA, Skudlarski P, et al: Gambling urges in pathological gambling: a functional magnetic resonance imaging study. Arch Gen Psychiatry 60:828–836, 2003

Robins E, Guze S: Establishment of diagnostic validity in psychiatric illness: its application to schizophrenia. Am J Psychiatry 126:983–987, 1970

Rose G: The Strategy of Preventive Medicine. New York, Oxford University Press, 1992

Tsuang M, Faraone S: The future of psychiatric genetics. Curr Psychiatr Rep 2:133–136, 2000

U.S. Department of Energy Human Genome Program: Beyond the Human Genome Project: what's next?, in Genomics and Its Impact on Science and Society: The Human Genome Project and Beyond. Washington, DC, U.S. Department of Energy Human Genome Program, 2003. Available at: http://www.ornl.gov/TechResources/Human_Genome/publicat/primer2001/5.html. Accessed September 6, 2003.

Winters KC, Rich T: A twin study of adult gambling behavior. J Gambl Stud 14: 213–225, 1999

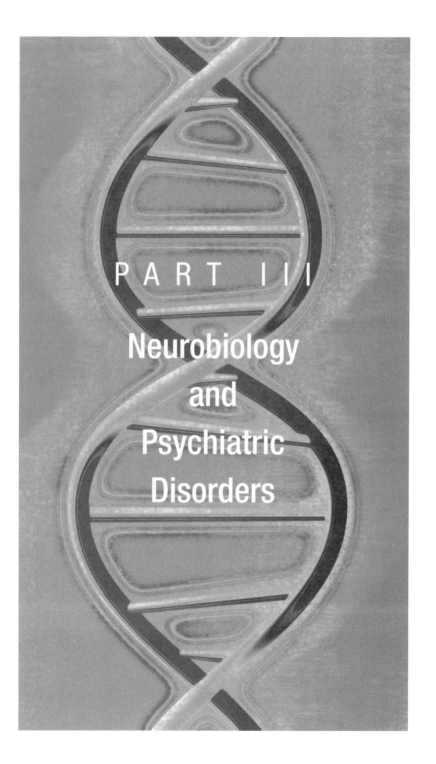

PART III

Neurobiology
and
Psychiatric
Disorders

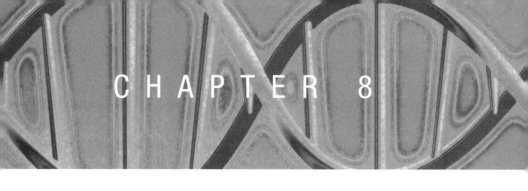

CHAPTER 8

Brain Structural Abnormalities in Mood Disorders

Wayne C. Drevets, M.D.

The recent development of neuroimaging technologies that permit in vivo quantitation of brain structural volumes enabled significant advances toward delineating the anatomical correlates of the affective disorders. Because these illnesses were not associated with gross brain pathology or with clear animal models for spontaneous, recurrent mood episodes, the availability of tools allowing noninvasive assessment of the human brain proved critical to illuminating the neurobiology of bipolar disorder and major depressive disorder (MDD). The results of imaging studies applying these technologies and of postmortem studies drawing on these neuroimaging data have guided clinical neuroscience toward models in which structural, as well as functional, brain pathology plays a role in the pathogenesis of mood disorders.

In many cases the discovery of structural brain abnormalities in mood disorders was facilitated by the results of longitudinal positron emission tomography (PET) imaging studies of MDD and bipolar disorder that identified abnormalities of regional cerebral glucose metabolism and cerebral blood flow (CBF) that persisted beyond symptom remission (reviewed in Drevets et al. 2004a; Figure 8–1). Some of the CBF and metabolic abnormalities evidenced during illness episodes proved to be mood state–dependent, presumably representing areas where changes

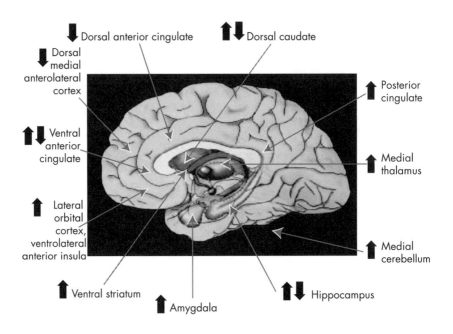

Dorsal anterior cingulate

Dorsal caudate

Dorsal medial anterolateral cortex

Posterior cingulate

Ventral anterior cingulate

Medial thalamus

Lateral orbital cortex, ventrolateral anterior insula

Medial cerebellum

Ventral striatum

Hippocampus

Amygdala

FIGURE 8–1.   Summary of neuropathological and morphometric changes (seen on neuroimaging) in early-onset primary major depressive disorder.

Arrows indicate direction of metabolic abnormality relative to control.

in metabolic activity reflected neurophysiological correlates of emotional and cognitive manifestations of the depressive syndrome (local glucose metabolism and CBF, which is tightly coupled to glucose metabolism, reflect summations of the energy utilization associated with terminal field synaptic transmission during neural activity [Magistretti and Pellerin 1999; Raichle 1987]). Others, however, persisted independently of mood state. This latter type of abnormality was hypothesized to reflect either neuropathological sequelae of recurrent illness or neuro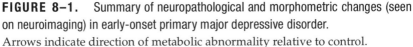developmental abnormalities that may confer vulnerability to MDD (e.g., in cases in which they were evident in otherwise healthy individuals at high familial risk for mood disorders). Such abnormalities in metabolism and CBF may be accounted for by pathological changes in synaptic transmission associated with alterations in neurotransmitter-receptor function, neuronal arborization/synapse formation, cellular proliferation, cerebrovascular function, or tissue volume (Links et al. 1996; Mazziotta et al. 1981; Wooten and Collins 1981). Several of the areas where metabolism and CBF appeared irreversibly *decreased* in individuals with

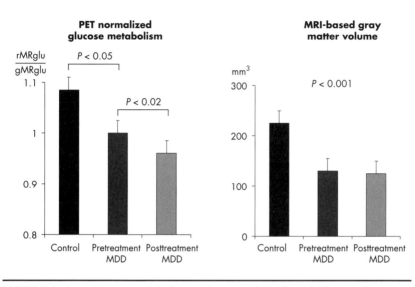

FIGURE 8–2. Glucose metabolism and gray matter volume in the anterior cingulate cortex in major depressive disorder (MDD).

Note. The reduction in subgenual anterior cingulate cortex (ACC) metabolism in depressed relative to control subjects appeared to be at least partly accounted for by a corresponding reduction in cortex volume on the left side (see text for details; Drevets et al. 1997). The bar histograms in the *left panel* of this figure show mean positron emission tomography (PET) normalized glucose metabolism for the left subgenual ACC measured using magnetic resonance imaging (MRI)–based region-of-interest analysis. Metabolism is decreased in the unmedicated MDD subjects relative to the healthy control subjects. In the same subject sample rescanned after a mean of 4 months of antidepressant drug treatment, metabolism was significantly lower than it had been in the unmedicated depressed condition (Drevets et al. 2002a). The *right panel* shows mean left subgenual ACC volume in the same subject sample measured using volumetric MRI. The volume is decreased in the unmedicated depressed subjects relative to the control subjects, and repeat MRI scans obtained at the time of the posttreatment PET scans show no differences in gray matter volume relative to the pretreatment MRI scan (Drevets et al. 1997). rMRgu = regional metabolic rate for glucose; gMRglu = global metabolic rate for glucose.

depression, relative to control subjects, were subsequently associated with focal tissue reductions in magnetic resonance imaging (MRI)–based morphometric and postmortem histopathological studies of MDD and bipolar disorder (e.g., Figure 8–2; Drevets et al. 1997, 1998; Mazziotta et al. 1981; Öngür et al. 1998).

The regions affected by these abnormalities have been shown to play major roles in modulating emotional behavior by electrophysiological, lesion analysis, and functional neuroimaging studies in healthy humans and experimental animals, suggesting that the structural abnormalities affecting these regions may give rise to dysregulation of mood and affect.

VOLUMETRIC MAGNETIC RESONANCE IMAGING ABNORMALITIES IN MOOD DISORDERS

The effect sizes of neuroimaging abnormalities discovered in mood disorders have been relatively small, such that the sensitivity for detecting them proved dependent upon technical issues of image acquisition and experimental design issues related to subject selection (reviewed in Drevets et al. 2004a). The major technical issues influencing sensitivity for detecting neuroimaging abnormalities in mood disorders hinge on the spatial and tissue contrast resolution of the image data. Volumetric resolution of state-of-the-art image data has recently been about 1 mm³, which compares with the cortex thickness of only 3–4 mm. MRI studies involving images of this resolution have been able to reproducibly show regionally specific reductions in mean gray matter volume across groups of clinically similar individuals with depression versus control subjects, although they lacked sensitivity for detecting the relatively subtle tissue reductions extant in mood disorders either in individual subjects or in small structures (e.g., amygdala). In contrast, studies attempting to replicate findings from such studies using data acquired at lower spatial resolutions (i.e., voxel sizes≥1.5 mm³) have commonly been negative, presumably because of the substantial partial volume effects associated with segmenting gray matter of only 3–4 mm cortex thickness in such low-resolution MRI images.

In other cases, disagreements within the literature may reflect differences in subject selection criteria, because the conditions encompassed by the diagnostic criteria for MDD appear heterogeneous with respect to pathophysiology and etiology. Notably, neuroimaging laboratories selecting depressed subjects according to the MDD criteria alone have rarely been able to replicate their own previous findings in independent subject samples. Instead, neuroimaging abnormalities appear specific to subsets of MDD subjects selected according to clinical characteristics such as familial aggregation of illness, age at illness onset, and capacity for developing mania or psychosis. For example, elderly MDD subjects with a late age at depression onset show an elevated prevalence of MRI signal hyperintensities in T_1-weighted MRI scans, which constitute putative correlates of cerebrovascular disease in this clinical setting in the deep and periventricular white matter relative both to elderly depressed persons with an early age at depression onset and age-matched, healthy control subjects. Similarly, MDD patients with either a late-life illness onset or delusions show lateral ventricle enlargement, a finding that generally has been absent in MDD patients who are elderly but have an early age of onset or are not delusional. As another example, third ventricle enlargement has been consistently reported in bipolar disorder, but not in MDD.

Frontal Lobe Structures

Volumes of the whole brain and entire frontal lobe generally have not differed between depressed and healthy control samples. In contrast, volumetric abnormalities have been identified in specific prefrontal cortical, basal ganglia, and mesiotemporal structures in affective disorders. The most prominent reductions of cortex were identified in the anterior cingulate cortex (ACC) ventral to the genu of the corpus callosum, where gray matter volume was abnormally decreased by 20%–40% in depressed subjects with familial pure depressive disease, familial bipolar disorder, or psychotic depression relative either to healthy control subjects or to mood-disordered subjects without affective-disordered first-degree relatives (Botteron et al. 2002; Drevets et al. 1997; Hirayasu et al. 1999). These findings were confirmed by postmortem studies of clinically similar samples. Treatment with selective serotonin reuptake inhibitors did not alter subgenual prefrontal cortex (PFC) volumes in MDD (Drevets et al. 1997), although this cortex was significantly larger in subjects with bipolar disorder who were chronically medicated with lithium or divalproex compared with bipolar subjects who were either unmedicated or medicated with other agents (Drevets et al. 2004a). These data appeared consistent with evidence that chronic administration of these mood stabilizers increases expression of the neurotrophic factors in rodents (Manji et al. 2001).

In the posterior orbital cortex and ventrolateral PFC volume also has been reduced in in vivo volumetric MRI studies (Bremner et al. 2002; Lai et al. 2000) and postmortem neuropathological studies of MDD (Bowen et al. 1989; Rajkowska et al. 1999). Reductions in gray matter volume also were found in the frontal polar/dorsal anterolateral PFC in MDD adults versus control subjects (Bell et al. 1999) and in adolescents with bipolar disorder versus control subjects (Dickstein et al. 2004) in post-mortem studies of MDD and bipolar disorder that reported abnormal reductions in the size of neurons and/or the density of glia (Cotter et al. 2001b; Rajkowska et al. 1999; Uranova et al. 2004).

Temporal Lobe Structures

Volumetric MRI (vMRI) studies of specific temporal lobe structures reported significant reductions in the hippocampal volume in MDD, with magnitudes of difference ranging from 8% to 19% with respect to healthy control subjects (e.g., Bremner et al. 2000; MacQueen et al. 2003; Mervaala et al. 2000; Nugent et al. 2004; Sheline et al. 1996, 1999; Steffens et al. 2000). Sheline et al. (1996) and MacQueen et al. (2003) reported that hippocampal volumes were negatively correlated with time spent depressed or with number of depressive episodes in MDD. Other groups found no differences in hippocampal volume between MDD and control samples (Ashtari et al. 1999; Axelson et al. 1993; Hauser et al. 1989; Pantel et al. 1997; Shah et al. 1998; Vakili et al. 2000; von Gunten et al. 2000). The inconsistency in the results of MDD studies may reflect biological heterogeneity within the subject samples. Vythilingam et al. (2002) found that hippocampal volume was abnormally decreased in depressed women who had suffered early life trauma, but not in women who had depression without early life trauma.

In bipolar disorder patients, hippocampal volume was reported by Swayze et al. (1992) and Noga et al. (2001) to be abnormally decreased; however, Pearlson et al. (1997) and Nugent et al. (2004) found that the hippocampal volume did not differ in comparison with healthy control subjects. In postmortem studies of patients with bipolar disorder, abnormal reductions in the mRNA concentrations of synaptic proteins (Eastwood and Harrison 2000) and in the apical dendritic spines of pyramidal neurons (Rosoklija et al. 2000) specifically were observed in the subiculum and ventral CA1 subregions of the hippocampus. A recent study conducted using high-resolution 3-tesla (3T) MRI found that the volume of the subiculum, but not the remainder of the hippocampus, was decreased in bipolar disorder patients relative to control subjects (Nugent et al. 2004).

The literature is in disagreement regarding the amygdala. In MDD patients, the amygdala volume was reported to be decreased (Sheline et al. 1998; Siegle et al. 2003), increased (Frodl et al. 2002), or not different (Mervaala et al. 2000) in comparison with the volume in healthy control subjects. In patients with bipolar disorder, the amygdala volume was similarly reported to be increased (Altshuler et al. 1998; Brambilla et al. 2003; Strakowski et al. 1999), decreased (Blumberg et al. 2003; DelBello et al. 2004; Pearlson et al. 1997), or not different (Swayze et al. 1992) compared with the volume in healthy control subjects. Although the extent to which disagreements in the results across studies are accounted for by confounding factors such as medication effects remains unclear, it appears more likely that MRI images acquired at 1.5 tesla or lower lack the spatial and tissue contrast resolution needed to measure the amygdala volume with sufficient validity and reliability. The amygdala's small size and proximity to other gray matter structures seriously limits accuracy for delimiting amygdala boundaries in images acquired using MRI scanners of 1.5 tesla or lower field strength.

High-resolution MRI scans acquired at 3-tesla magnetic field strength, in contrast, permit valid and reliable measures of amygdala volume. A recent study employing this technique established that amygdala volume is decreased bilaterally both in currently depressed and currently remitted MDD subjects compared with healthy control subjects (Drevets et al. 2004b). Although mean amygdala volumes did not differ between bipolar disorder patients and control samples in this study, they were smaller in bipolar disorder subjects who had not been medicated recently with mood stabilizers than in those who had been taking such agents, consistent with evidence that some mood stabilizers exert neurotrophic effects (Manji et al. 2001).

Basal Ganglia

Volumes of some basal ganglia structures also were reported to be abnormal in affective disorders. Husain et al. (1991) reported that the putamen was smaller in patients with depression (mean age, 55 years) than in control subjects, and Krishnan et al. (1992) found the caudate nucleus to be smaller in those with depression (mean age, 48 years) than in control subjects. In elderly depressed patients, Krishnan et al. (1993) also found smaller putamen and caudate volumes relative to control subjects. These findings were consistent with the postmortem study of Baumann et al. (1999), which found that caudate and accumbens area volumes were decreased in MDD and bipolar disorder samples compared with control samples. Nevertheless, Dupont et al. (1995) and Lenze et al. (1999) failed to find significant differences in caudate or lentiform nucleus (putamen plus pallidum) volumes between younger MDD subjects and control subjects.

Corpus Callosum

The genual subsection of the corpus callosum was reduced in volume both in adults with MDD and in never-depressed female offspring of mothers with MDD (Brambilla et al. 2004; Martinez et al. 2002). These white-matter regions contain transcallosal fibers connecting the orbital cortex, ACC, and medial PFC with their homologous cortices in the contralateral hemisphere. Volumes of the splenial subregion of the corpus callosum, which contains transcallosal fibers from the posterior cingulate cortex, also were decreased in mood disordered versus control samples.

Other Cerebral Structures

vMRI studies of other brain structures in mood disorders have produced less consistent results. Of vMRI studies of the thalamus, Dupont et al. (1995) reported the volume of the thalamus was decreased in MDD subjects compared with control samples, but Krishnan et al. (1991a, 1993) found no differences between those with depression and control subjects. Two vMRI studies of the thalamus in bipolar disorder also reported conflicting results. Of MRI studies of the cerebellum, two found that vermal volume was reduced in MDD subjects relative to control subjects (Escalona et al. 1993; Shah et al. 1992), whereas a third study that employed computed tography scanning did not find evidence of global cerebellar atrophy (Yates et al. 1987).

Consistent with evidence that the function of the hypothalamic-pituitary-adrenal axis is elevated in some subjects with affective disorders, enlargement of the pituitary and adrenal glands has been reported in MDD. Krishnan et al. (1991b) found that the cross-sectional area and volume of the pituitary were increased 34% and 41%, respectively, in depressed subjects relative to control subjects. This observation was consistent with evidence that the adrenal gland also is abnormally enlarged in MDD (for review, see Drevets et al. 2004a), putatively reflecting excessive stimulation of the adrenal cortex by adrenocorticotropic hormone.

POSTMORTEM NEUROPATHOLOGICAL ASSESSMENTS OF MOOD DISORDERS

Most regions in which MRI studies demonstrated volumetric abnormalities in mood disorders also were found to contain histopathological changes or gray matter volumetric reductions in postmortem studies of

MDD and bipolar disorder (Table 8–1). Reductions in gray matter volume, thickness, or wet weight were reported in the subgenual ACC, posterolateral orbital cortex, and ventral striatum in MDD and/or bipolar disorder subjects relative to control subjects (Baumann et al. 1999; Bowen et al. 1989; Drevets et al. 1998; Öngür et al. 1998; Rajkowska et al. 1999). The histopathological correlates of these abnormalities included reductions in glial cells with no equivalent loss of neurons, reductions in synapses or synaptic proteins, elevations in neuron density, and reductions in neuron size (Bowen et al. 1989; Cotter et al. 2000, 2001b; Eastwood and Harrison 2000, 2001; Öngür et al. 1998; Rajkowska et al. 1999). Abnormal reductions in glial cell counts and density and in glial cell-to-neuron ratios also have been found in MDD in the pregenual ACC (Brodmann area [BA] 24; Cotter et al. 2001b), the frontal polar/dorsal anterolateral PFC (BA 9; Cotter et al. 2002; Uranova et al. 2004), and the amygdala (Bowley et al. 2002; Hamidi et al. 2004). Finally, the mean size of neurons was reduced in the dorsal anterolateral PFC (BA 9) in MDD subjects relative to control subjects (Rajkowska et al. 1999), and the density of neurons was decreased in the ACC in bipolar disorder (Benes et al. 2001). In most studies, the decreases largely were accounted for by differences involving the left hemisphere (Bowen et al. 1989; Bowley et al. 2002; Drevets et al. 1998; Hamidi et al. 2004; Öngür et al. 1998).

In the amygdala and dorsal anterolateral PFC (BA 9), the glial cell type that differed between MDD and control samples was the oligodendrocyte. In contrast, astrocyte and microglial cell counts in the amygdala did not differ significantly between MDD or bipolar disorder subjects and healthy control subjects (Hamidi et al. 2004). Oligodendroglia are best characterized for their role in myelination, and the reduction in oligodendrocytes may conceivably arise secondary to an effect on myelin, either through demyelination, abnormal development, or atrophy in the number of myelinated axons. Notably, the myelin basic protein concentration was decreased in the frontal polar cortex (BA 10) in MDD subjects (Honer et al. 1999). Compatible with these data, the concentration of white matter in the vicinity of the amygdala (A.C. Nugent, W.C. Drevets, unpublished data, 2005) and the volume of white matter in the genual and splenial portions of the corpus callosum were abnormally reduced in MDD and bipolar disorder (Brambilla et al. 2004; Martinez et al. 2002). These corpus callosal subregions were also smaller in never-depressed child and adolescent offspring of women with MDD, relative to control subjects, suggesting this reduction in white matter may reflect a developmental deficit that exists before the onset of depressive episodes (Martinez et al. 2002). These observations also support the hypothesis

TABLE 8–1. Histopathological changes found in mood disorders

Region	Glial markers	Synaptic markers	Interneurons	Pyramidal cells
Dorsolateral prefrontal cortex (BA 9)	↓			↓ MDD
Subgenual anterior cingulate cortex	↓	↓		
Pregenual anterior cingulate cortex	↓	↓	↓ Bipolar disorder	
Orbital cortex	↓ Caudal			↓ Rostral
Ventrolateral prefrontal cortex	↓			
Frontal polar cortex (BA 10)	↓ Bipolar disorder			
Amygdala	↓ MDD			
Caudate	↓ Bipolar disorder			
Hippocampus		↓ Bipolar disorder	↓ Bipolar disorder	

Note. MDD=major depressive disorder.

that the glial cell loss in mood disorders is accounted for by a reduction in myelinating oligodendrocytes.

Also supportive of this hypothesis are reports that the reductions in glia in mood disorders depended on laminar analysis, with the greatest effects in layers III, V, and VI (Cotter et al. 2001b, 2002; Rajkowska et al. 1999, 2001). The intracortical plexi of myelinated axons known as "bands of Baillarger" are generally concentrated in layers III and V. The size of these plexi varies across cortical areas, so if the oligodendrocytes related to these plexi were affected, different areas would show greater or lesser deficits. Layer VI in particular has a relatively large component of myelinated fibers running between the gray and white matter.

Finally, a population of satellite oligodendrocytes exists adjacent to neuron cell bodies that do not appear to have a role in myelination under normal conditions (Ludwin 1984) and instead may play a role in maintaining the extracellular environment for neurons that resembles the functions mediated by astrocytes. For example, satellite oligodendrocytes are immunohistochemically reactive for glutamine synthetase, suggesting they function like astrocytes to take up synaptically released glutamate for conversion to glutamine and cycling back into neurons (D'Amelio et al. 1990). Many studies of glial function have not distinguished astrocytes from oligodendrocytes, and the two glial types may share multiple functions. An electron microscopy study of the PFC in bipolar disorder revealed decreased nuclear size, clumping of chromatin, and other types of damage to satellite oligodendrocytes, providing evidence of both apoptotic and necrotic degeneration (Uranova et al. 2001). Fewer signs of degeneration were observed in myelinating oligodendrocytes in white matter.

In other brain regions, reductions in astroglia were reported by postmortem studies of affective disorders. In the frontal cortex, Johnston-Wilson et al. (2000) found that four forms of the astrocytic product glial fibrillary acidic protein (GFAP) were decreased in mood-disordered subjects relative to control subjects, although it remained unclear whether this decrement reflected a reduction in astrocyte density or a reduction in GFAP expression. Using immunohistochemical staining for GFAP, Webster et al. (2001) found no differences in cortical astrocytes among the MDD, bipolar disorder, and control groups. Other studies also did not find differences in GFAP between the mood disorder sample and control sample (for review, see Cotter et al. 2001a).

ASSOCIATION BETWEEN STRUCTURAL AND METABOLIC ABNORMALITIES

Factors that may conceivably contribute to a loss of oligodendroglia in mood disorders include the putative elevations of glucocorticoid secretion and glutamatergic transmission evident during depression (and possibly during mania as well). Glucocorticoids affect glia as well as neurons (Cheng and de Vellis 2000), and elevated glucocorticoid levels decrease the proliferation of oligodendroglial precursors (Alonso 2000).

Moreover, oligodendrocytes express AMPA (α-amino-3-hydroxy-5-methyl-4-isoxazole propionic acid) and kainate type glutamate receptors and are sensitive to excitotoxic damage (e.g., from excess glutamate) and to oxidative stress (reviewed in Hamidi et al. 2004). These vulnerabilities putatively contribute to oligodendrocyte degeneration in ischemic brain injury and demyelinating diseases (Dewar et al. 2003; Matute et al. 1997), although no data exist to establish a similar role in affective disorders. The targeted nature of the reductions in gray matter volume and in glial cells to specific areas within limbic-cortical circuits where glucose metabolism is elevated during depression is noteworthy in light of evidence that regional glucose metabolism predominantly reflects local glutamatergic transmission. The hypothesis that glutamate transmission is elevated in these areas in depression is supported by the postmortem study by Nowak et al. (1995) in depressed suicide victims.

Elevations of glutamate transmission and cortisol secretion in mood disorders also may contribute to reductions in gray matter volume and synaptic markers by inducing dendritic atrophy in specific brain regions. In the medial PFC and parts of the hippocampus and amygdala of adult rodents, the dendritic arbors undergo atrophy and debranching in response to repeated or chronic stress (McEwen and Magarinos 2001). The effects of stress on dendritic arborization depend on both the type of stress applied and the anatomical location under investigation. For example, chronic, unpredictable stress produces dendritic atrophy in the basolateral amygdala, whereas chronic immobilization stress increased dendritic branching in pyramidal and stellate neurons of the basolateral amygdala but did not alter dendritic arborization in the amygdala central nucleus (Vyas et al. 2002, 2003). These dendritic reshaping processes depend on interactions between the elevated N-methyl-D-aspartate (NMDA) receptor stimulation and glucocorticoid secretion associated with repeated stress (McEwen and Magarinos 2001).

Depressed individuals with bipolar disorder and MDD who show regional reductions in gray matter volume also show evidence of having increased cortisol secretion and glutamate transmission. Specifically, depressed subjects with familial pure depressive disease (FPDD) or bipolar disorder are more likely to show abnormal suppression of cortisol secretion by dexamethasone and blunted hypoglycemic response to insulin (reviewed in Drevets et al. 2002c) and to release excessive amounts of cortisol during stress (Drevets et al. 1999, 2002a, 2002c). Subjects with FPDD or familial bipolar disorder also show elevations of glucose metabolism in the medial and orbital PFC, amygdala, ventral striatum, and ACC regions where gray matter volume and cellular elements are abnormally decreased.

The glucose metabolic signal is dominated by changes in glutamate transmission, so the specificity of gray matter reductions to regions where glucose metabolism is elevated during depression raises the possibility that excitatory amino acid transmission plays a role in the neuropathology of mood disorders. At least 85%–90% of the glucose metabolic signal is accounted for by glutamate transmission (Magistretti and Pellerin 1999; Rothman et al. 1999; Shen et al. 1999; Shulman and Rothman 1998; Sibson et al. 1998). In the depressed phase of familial MDD and bipolar disorder, glucose metabolism and CBF are abnormally increased in the amygdala, lateral orbital/ventrolateral PFC, ACC anterior to the genu of the corpus callosum ("pregenual" ACC), posterior cingulate cortex, ventral striatum, medial thalamus, and medial cerebellum (for review, see Drevets et al. 2004). During effective antidepressant drug or electroconvulsive therapy, metabolic activity decreases in all of these regions (for review, see Drevets et al. 2002a, 2004a), potentially consistent with evidence that these treatments result in desensitization of NMDA-glutamatergic receptors in the frontal cortex of rodents. In addition to these areas of increased glucose metabolism, areas of reduced metabolism in depressed versus control subjects were found in the subgenual ACC (Drevets et al. 1997) and the dorsal medial/dorsal anterolateral PFC (Baxter et al. 1989; Bell et al. 1999; Bench et al. 1992). Yet even in these regions, metabolic activity increases during depressive relapse induced by tryptophan depletion (which depletes central serotonin transmission; see Neumeister et al. 2004a), and metabolism is increased in the subgenual ACC in the unmedicated-depressed phase relative to the medicated-remitted phase. In regions where metabolism is increased in the depressed relative to the remitted phase of MDD, reductions in cortex volume and/or histopathological changes consistently have been found in in vivo MRI studies and/or postmortem studies of MDD.

The hypothesis that the elevations in glucose metabolism seen in these circuits reflect elevations in glutamatergic transmission is supported by evidence that the anatomical projections between affected areas are excitatory in nature. The abnormal increases in CBF and metabolism in the ventrolateral and orbital PFC, ventral ACC, amygdala, ventral striatum, and medial thalamus evident in depression implicate a limbic-thalamo-cortical circuit involving the amygdala, mediodorsal nucleus of the thalamus, and orbital and medial PFC and a limbic-striatal-pallidal-thalamic circuit involving related parts of the striatum and ventral pallidum along with the components of the other circuit (Drevets et al. 1992). The first of these circuits can be conceptualized as an excitatory triangular circuit whereby the basolateral amygdala and the orbital and medial PFC are interconnected by excitatory (largely glutamatergic) projections with each other and the mediodorsal nucleus (Amaral and Insausti 1992; Drevets et al. 1992; Jackson and Moghaddam 2001; Kuroda and Price 1991; Matsuda and Fujimura 1995; McDonald 1994; Rainnie et al. 1991; Velasco et al. 1989), so increased metabolic activity in these structures would presumably reflect increased synaptic transmission through the limbic-thalamo-cortical circuit. The limbic-striatal-pallidal-thalamic circuit constitutes a disinhibitory side loop between the amygdala or

PFC and the mediodorsal nucleus. The amygdala and PFC send excitatory projections to overlapping parts of the ventromedial striatum. This part of the striatum sends an inhibitory projection to the ventral pallidum (Graybiel 1990) which in turn sends GABAergic inhibitory fibers to the mediodorsal nucleus (Kuroda and Price 1991).

IMPLICATIONS FOR THE PATHOGENESIS OF EMOTION DYSREGULATION

The circuits just described also have been implicated in depressive syndromes arising secondary to lesions or degenerative illnesses. Lesions involving the PFC (i.e., tumors or infarctions) and the diseases of the basal ganglia (e.g., Parkinson's or Huntington's disease) that are associated with higher rates of depression, compared with other similarly debilitating conditions, result in dysfunction at distinct points within these circuits and affect synaptic transmission in diverse ways (for review, see Drevets and Todd, in press). Consistent with this hypothesis, imaging studies of depressive syndromes arising secondary to neurological disorders generally show results that differ from those obtained in primary mood disorders. In contrast to the elevations of CBF and metabolism in the orbital cortex in persons with primary depression, for example, flow in this region is decreased or not significantly different in subjects with depressive syndromes arising secondary to Parkinson's disease, Huntington's disease, or basal ganglia infarction compared with nondepressed control subjects with the same illnesses (Mayberg et al. 1990, 1991, 1992; Ring et al. 1994). Primary and secondary depressive syndromes are thus likely to involve the same neural network, although the pattern of altered synaptic transmission and the direction of physiological abnormalities within individual structures may differ across conditions. One common substrate in these cases may impair prefrontal cortical-striatal modulation of limbic and visceral functions, because both the idiopathic, neuropathological changes seen in the orbital and medial PFC and the ventral striatum in primary mood disorders and the distinct neuropathologies associated with neurodegenerative conditions appear capable of inducing depressive syndromes (e.g., Parkinson's disease, Huntington's disease, cerebrovascular disease).

Prefrontal cortical-amygdalar projections also may play a role in the pathogenesis of depressive and anxiety symptoms in mood disorders. Although the reciprocal prefrontal cortical-amygdalar projections are excitatory in nature, these connections ultimately appear to activate inhibitory interneurons that in turn lead to functional inhibition in the projected field of the amygdala (for PFC-to-amygdalar projections) or the PFC (for reviews, see Amaral and Insausti 1992; Drevets 2003; Garcia et al. 1999; Jackson and Moghaddam 2001; Matsuda and Fujimura 1995; McDonald 1994; Perez-Jaranay and Vives 1991; Rainnie et al. 1991; Rosenkranz and Grace 2002; Velasco et al. 1989). The function of the PFC in modulating the amygdala appears impaired in mood disorders, as evident from functional MRI data showing that abnormally sustained amygdala activity in response to aversive words or sad faces in MDD is associated with blunted activation of anatomically related PFC areas (Drevets 2003; Siegle et al. 2002). Thus, the volumetric and/or histopathological changes evident in the subgenual and pregenual ACC, lateral orbital cortex, dorsomedial/dorsal anterolateral PFC, hippocampal subiculum, amygdala, and ventral striatum may interfere with the modulation of emotional behavior, as discussed later.

Ventral Anterior Cingulate Cortex

The ACC ventral and anterior to the genu of the corpus callosum (subgenual and pregenual, respectively) shows complex relationships between metabolism and illness state, which appear accounted for by a left-lateralized reduction of the corresponding cortex, initially demonstrated by vMRI-based morphometric measures (Botteron et al. 2002; Buchsbaum et al. 1997; Drevets et al. 1997; Hirayasu et al. 1999) and later by postmortem studies of familial bipolar disorder and MDD (Öngür et al. 1998). Thus, computer simulations that correct the PET data acquired in this region for the partial volume averaging effect associated with the reduction in gray matter volume measured in vMRI scans from the same subjects conclude that the actual metabolic activity in the remaining subgenual PFC tissue is *increased* in depressed compared with control subjects and decreases to normative levels during treatment (Drevets 1999) (Figure 8–2). This conclusion was noteworthy in light of evidence that effective antidepressant pharmacotherapy resulted in a *decrease* in metabolic activity in this region in MDD (Buchsbaum et al. 1997; Drevets et al. 2002a, 2002b; Mayberg et al. 1999), that during depressive episodes metabolism correlated positively with depression severity (Drevets et al. 2002a, 2002b; Osuch et al. 2000), and that flow increased in this region in healthy, nondepressed humans during experimentally induced sadness (Damasio et al. 2000; George et al. 1995; Mayberg et al. 1999).

The reduction in volume in this region exists early in the illness in familial bipolar disorder (Hirayasu et al. 1999) and MDD (Botteron et al. 2002). Nevertheless, preliminary evidence in twins discordant for MDD that showed that the affected twin had a smaller volume than the un-affected co-twin (Botteron et al. 1999) suggested that this gray matter deficit may be initiated or worsened by depressive episodes. Kimbrell et al. (2002) reported that the subgenual ACC metabolism correlated inversely with the number of lifetime depressive episodes, compatible with the possibility that the metabolic reduction measured with PET reflects a gray matter reduction that worsens with repeated illness.

In the pregenual ACC, Drevets et al. (1992) found increased CBF in MDD, and subsequent studies extended this observation by demonstrating complex relationships between pregenual ACC activity and treatment outcome. Wu et al. (1992) reported that depressed persons whose mood improved during sleep deprivation showed elevated metabolism in the pregenual ACC and amygdala in their pretreatment, baseline scans. Mayberg et al. (1997) reported that although metabolism in the pregenual ACC was abnormally increased in depressed subjects who subsequently responded to antidepressant drugs, metabolism was decreased in those who later had poor treatment response. Finally, in a tomographic electroencephalogram analysis, Pizzagalli et al. (2001) reported that depressed subjects who ultimately showed the best response to nortriptyline showed hyperactivity (higher theta activity) in the pregenual ACC in the pretreatment, baseline condition compared with subjects showing poorer responses. During antidepressant treatment, most PET studies have shown that pregenual ACC metabolism and CBF decrease in post- relative to pretreatment scans (reviewed in Drevets et al. 2004a). The finding that histopathological changes occur in this region in MDD and bipolar disorder (Benes et al. 2001; Cotter et al. 2000, 2001b) suggests that the abnormal reduction in metabolism in those with treatment-resistant illness may reflect more severe reductions in cortex.

In rodents and nonhuman primates, the cortical areas that appear homologous to human subgenual and pregenual ACC—namely, the infralimbic, prelimbic, and ventral ACCs—have extensive anatomical connections with areas implicated in the expression of autonomic, endocrine, and behavioral responses to threat or stress, such as the amygdala, lateral hypothalamus, periaqueductal gray, accumbens, subiculum, orbital cortex, ventral tegmental area, raphe, locus coeruleus, and nucleus tractus solitarius (Drevets et al. 1998; Öngür and Price 2000). Humans with lesions that include the subgenual and pregenual ACC show abnormal autonomic responses to emotionally provocative stimuli and inability to experience emotion related to concepts that ordinarily evoke emotion (Damasio 1995). Electrical stimulation of the ACC elicits fear, panic, or a sense of foreboding in humans and vocalization in experi-

mental animals (reviewed in Price et al. 1996). Similarly, rats with experimental lesions of prelimbic cortex demonstrate altered autonomic, neuroendocrine, and behavioral responses to stress and fear-conditioned
stimuli. The prelimbic and infralimbic cortices contain abundant concentrations of glucocorticoid receptors that, when stimulated by corticosterone, reduce glucocorticoid responses to stress (Dioro et al. 1993).
Lesions of these cortices consequently result in exaggerated adrenocorticotropic hormone and corticosterone secretion during restraint stress
(Dioro et al. 1993). In rats, bilateral or *right*-lateralized lesions of the infralimbic, prelimbic, and anterior cingulate cortices attenuate sympathetic
autonomic responses, stress-induced corticosterone secretion, and gastric
stress pathology during restraint stress or exposure to fear-conditioned
stimuli (Frysztak and Neafsey 1994; Morgan and LeDoux 1995; Sullivan
and Gratton 1999). In contrast, *left*-sided lesions of this area increase
sympathetic autonomic arousal and corticosterone responses to restraint
stress (Sullivan and Gratton 1999). These data suggest the right subgenual
PFC facilitates visceral responses during emotional processing, whereas
the left subgenual PFC inhibits or modulates such responses (Sullivan
and Gratton 1999). Notably the gray matter reduction in this region in
MDD and bipolar disorder was left lateralized, suggesting it may contribute to disinhibition of neuroendocrine responses and dysregulation
of autonomic function in depression (Carney et al. 1993; Dioro et al. 1993;
Veith et al. 1994).

The ventral ACC also participates in neural processing related to behavioral incentive and motivated behavior. These areas send efferent
projections to the ventral tegmental area and substantia nigra and receive dense dopaminergic innervation from the former (Öngür and Price
2000). In rats, glutamatergic or electrical stimulation of medial PFC areas that include the prelimbic cortex elicits burst firing patterns from
ventral tegmental area dopaminergic cells and increases dopamine release in the accumbens (for review, see Drevets 1999). These phasic, burst
firing patterns of dopaminergic neurons appear to encode information regarding stimuli that predict reward as well as deviations between such
predictions and actual experience of reward (Schultz 1997). Ventral ACC
dysfunction may thus conceivably contribute to disturbances of he-
donic perception and motivated behavior in affective disorders.

Dorsomedial/Dorsal Anterolateral Prefrontal Cortex

Metabolism is abnormally decreased in the dorsolateral and dorsomedial PFC in MDD (for review, see Drevets et al. 2004a). The dorsomedial

PFC region includes the dorsal ACC (Bench et al. 1992) and the cortex rostral to the dorsal ACC lying on the medial and lateral surfaces of the superior frontal gyrus (BA 9 and possibly BA 32; Baxter et al. 1989; Bell et al. 1999; Drevets et al. 2002a). Postmortem studies of MDD and bipolar disorder found abnormal reductions in the size of neurons and/or the density of glia in this portion of BA 9 (Cotter et al. 2001b; Orlovskaya et al. 2000; Rajkowska et al. 1999), which may account for the metabolic deficit in this region and for the failure of antidepressant drug treatment to correct metabolism in these areas in MDD (Bell et al. 1999; Drevets et al. 2002a). Nevertheless, remitted MDD subjects who experience depressive relapse during tryptophan depletion show an increase in metabolic activity in these areas in the depressed versus the remitted conditions (Neumeister et al. 2004b), similar to the pattern that occurs in other structures where histopathological and gray matter volume changes exist in MDD.

Normally CBF increases in the dorsomedial/dorsal anterolateral PFC in healthy humans as they perform tasks that elicit emotional responses or require emotional evaluations (reviewed in Drevets et al. 2004a). For example, during anxious anticipation of an electrical shock, CBF increases in this region in healthy humans, and the magnitude of the hemodynamic response correlates inversely with changes in anxiety ratings and heart rate. This behavioral correlation suggests that this region functions to attenuate emotional expression, potentially compatible with evidence that rats with lesions of the dorsomedial PFC show exaggerated heart rate responses to fear-conditioned stimuli and that stimulation of these sites in rats attenuates defensive behavior and cardiovascular responses evoked by amygdala stimulation (reviewed in Frysztak and Neafsey 1994; although the homologue to these areas in primates has not been clearly established). In primates the BA 9 cortex sends efferent projections to the lateral periaqueductal gray and the dorsal hypothalamus through which it may modulate cardiovascular responses associated with emotional behavior (Öngür and Price 2000). Dysfunction of the dorsomedial/dorsal anterolateral PFC may thus conceivably interfere with the modulation of emotional responses in affective disorders.

Lateral Orbital/Ventrolateral Prefrontal Cortex

In the lateral orbital cortex, ventrolateral PFC, and anterior insula, metabolism is abnormally increased in unmedicated subjects with primary MDD (reviewed in Drevets et al. 2004). The elevated activity in these areas in MDD appears mood state dependent (Drevets et al. 1992), and metabolism and CBF decrease in these regions during somatic antidepressant treatments (for review, see Drevets et al. 2004). The relationship between depression severity and physiological activity in the lateral orbital cortex/ventrolateral PFC is complex. Metabolism and CBF increase in these areas in the depressed relative to the remitted phases of MDD, yet are inversely correlated with ratings of depressive ideation and severity (Drevets et al. 1992, 1995a, 2002b). Moreover, although metabolism is abnormally increased in these areas in depressed patients with treatment-responsive MDD or bipolar disorder, more severely ill patients or those with treatment-refractory illness show CBF and metabolic values lower than or not different from those of control subjects (Mayberg et al. 1994, 1997). These inverse relationships between orbital cortex/ventrolateral PFC metabolism and depression severity also extend to other emotional states. For example, posterior orbital cortex CBF increases in subjects with obsessive-compulsive disorder or simple animal phobias during exposure to phobic stimuli and in healthy subjects during induced sadness (Drevets et al. 1995b; Rauch et al. 1994; Schneider et al. 1995) to an extent that is inversely correlated with changes in obsessive thinking, anxiety, and sadness, respectively.

These data appear consistent with electrophysiological and lesion analysis data showing that parts of the orbital cortex participate in modulating visceral and behavioral responses associated with defensive, emotional, and reward-directed behavior as reinforcement contingencies change (Mogenson et al. 1993; Öngür and Price 2000; Rolls 1995). The orbital cortex and amygdala send overlapping projections to each other and to the ventral striatum, hypothalamus, and periaqueductal gray through which they appear to modulate each other's effects on emotional behavior (Mogenson et al. 1993; Öngür and Price 2000; Timms 1977).

Activation of the ventrolateral PFC/orbital cortex during depression may thus reflect compensatory attempts to attenuate emotional expression or interrupt aversive thought and emotion. Consistent with this hypothesis, cerebrovascular lesions of this cortex are associated with an increased risk for developing major depression (MacFall et al. 2001). Thus the reduction of CBF and metabolism in the orbital cortex and ventrolateral PFC during antidepressant drug treatment may not be a primary mechanism through which such agents ameliorate depressive symptoms. Instead, direct inhibition of pathological limbic activity in areas such as the amygdala and right subgenual ACC may attenuate the mediation of depressive symptoms (Drevets et al. 2002a). The orbital cortex neurons may thus relax, as reflected by the return of metabolism to normative levels, as antidepressant drug therapy attenuates limbic activity to which these neurons putatively respond (Garcia et al. 1999; Oya et al. 2001).

Amygdala

In the amygdala, physiological activity is altered, both at rest and during exposure to emotionally valenced stimuli in affective disorders. Elevated basal metabolism has been found in depressed subjects who meet criteria for FPDD (Figure 8–3; Drevets et al. 1992, 1995a, 2002a, 2002c), MDD-melancholic subtype (Nofzinger et al. 1999), type II bipolar disorder, or nonpsychotic type I bipolar disorder (Drevets et al. 2002c; Ketter et al. 2001) or those who prove responsive to sleep deprivation (Wu et al. 1992). In contrast, metabolism has not been shown to be abnormal in MDD subjects meeting criteria for depression spectrum disease (Drevets et al. 1995a, 2002c) or in MDD samples meeting DSM-IV-TR (American Psychiatric Association 2000) criteria for MDD as sole inclusion criterion (Abercrombie et al. 1998; Brody et al. 2001; Saxena et al. 2002), although the interpretation of the latter results was confounded by technical problems that reduced sensitivity for measuring amygdala activity (Drevets et al. 2002c).

Amygdala metabolism decreases toward normative levels during effective antidepressant drug treatment (Drevets et al. 2002a).

The hemodynamic response of the left amygdala was blunted in depressed children while they were viewing fearful faces (Thomas et al. 2001) and adults (Drevets 2001), consistent with the elevation of resting metabolism in this structure in MDD (physiologically activated tissue is expected to show attenuation of further rises in hemodynamic/metabolic signal in response to tasks that engage that tissue).

The duration of hemodynamic responses to sad stimuli, in particular, is also abnormal in depression. Drevets (2001) observed that although the initial amygdala CBF response to sad faces was similar in depressed and control subjects, this response habituated during repeated exposures to the same stimuli in control but not in depressed subjects over the imaging period. Siegle et al. (2002) found that hemodynamic activity increased in the amygdala during exposure to negatively valenced words to a similar extent in depressed and control subjects but that the hemodynamic response rapidly fell to baseline in the control subjects, while remaining elevated in those who were depressed.

The amygdala plays major roles in organizing autonomic, neuroendocrine, and behavioral aspects of emotional/stress responses to ex-

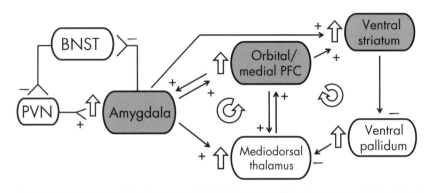

FIGURE 8–3. Anatomical circuits hypothesized to participate in the functional anatomy of major depressive disorder based on functional neuroimaging, lesion analysis, and postmortem neuropathological evidence.

Note. The monosynaptic connections among regions are illustrated (*closed arrows*), with "+" indicating excitatory (mainly glutamatergic) and "–" indicating inhibitory projections. The prefrontal cortex (PFC) areas referred to involve primarily the lateral orbital and ventrolateral PFC and ventral anterior cingulate cortex. The parts of the striatum under consideration are the ventral medial caudate and accumbens area, which particularly project to the ventral pallidum. The *open straight arrows* adjacent to each region indicate the direction of differences in glucose metabolism in the unmedicated-depressed phase relative to the treated-remitted phase of familial pure depressive disease. The findings of increased flow and metabolism in the amygdala, medial thalamus, and limbic PFC are compatible with other evidence suggesting that synaptic transmission through the limbic-thalamo-cortical circuit is abnormally elevated, as designated by the *curved arrow*. Because the metabolic signal predominantly reflects glutamatergic transmission, it is hypothesized that reverberatory excitatory transmission plays a role in the development of the reported reductions in gray matter in the amygdala, PFC, and ventral striatum in major depressive disorder (see text for details). PVN=paraventricular nucleus; BNST=bed nucleus of the stria terminalis.

periential stimuli. For example, the amygdala facilitates stress-related corticotropin-releasing hormone (CRH) release (Herman and Cullinan 1997), suggesting a mechanism by which excessive amygdala activity may participate in inducing the CRH and cortisol hypersecretion evident in MDD. The left amygdala metabolism specifically correlated positively with stressed plasma cortisol secretion in MDD and bipolar disorder, possibly reflecting the effect of amygdala activity on CRH secretion and/or the effect of cortisol and CRH on amygdala function (Drevets et al. 2002c).

If the reduction in amygdala volume is associated with reductions in synaptic contacts formed by afferent projections from cortical regions known to modulate amygdala function, then amygdala neuronal activity may become disinhibited (Garcia et al. 1999; Rosenkranz and Grace 2002). The previously cited reports that amygdala metabolism is abnormally elevated and that hemodynamic responses of the amygdala to emotional stimuli are abnormally persistent in MDD are compatible with this hypothesis. For example, Siegle et al. (2003) reported that the abnormally persistent hemodynamic responses of the amygdala to sad words occurred specifically in MDD subjects who had reduced amygdala volumes. If the neurotrophic effects of mood-stabilizing drugs protect and restore modulatory connections between the amygdala and cortex (Drevets et al. 2004b), then the volumetric increases observed during treatment may contribute to their therapeutic effects in affective disorders.

Abnormalities in Anatomically Related Limbic and Subcortical Structures

In the medial thalamus and ventral striatum, metabolism is abnormally elevated in the depressed phase of MDD and bipolar disorder and is decreased during antidepressant pharmacotherapy (Drevets et al. 1992, 1995a, 2002b; Saxena et al. 2002; Videbech et al. 2001; Wilson et al. 2002).

Metabolism and CBF also appear abnormally increased in the posterior cingulate cortex in unmedicated depressed subjects with MDD (e.g., Bench et al. 1993; Buchsbaum et al. 1997; Drevets et al. 2002a). Bench et al. (1993) specifically reported that posterior cingulate CBF correlated positively with anxiety ratings in MDD—a finding that is potentially consistent with observations that exposure to aversive stimuli of various types results in increased hemodynamic activity in the posterior cingulate cortex (reviewed in Charney and Drevets 2002).

NEURORECEPTOR IMAGING ABNORMALITIES IN MOOD DISORDERS

Receptor imaging studies of affective disorders have demonstrated reductions of serotonin type 1A (5-HT_{1A}) receptor binding that may hold major implications for alterations in neuroplasticity in these conditions. Both presynaptic (raphe nuclei) and postsynaptic (insula, anterior and posterior cingulate cortices, parieto-occipital cortex, orbital/ventrolateral

PFC) 5-HT$_{1A}$ receptor binding are abnormally decreased in MDD and panic disorder (irrespective of the presence of comorbid depression) and postsynaptic 5-HT$_{1A}$ receptor binding also is decreased in bipolar disorder (Bain et al. 2004; Drevets et al. 1999; Neumeister et al. 2004b; Parsey et al. 2002; Sargent et al. 2000). The magnitudes of these differences appear similar to those found in postmortem studies of primary mood disorders (Bowen et al. 1989; Lopez et al. 1998) or depressed suicide victims (Arango et al. 2001). These data also were compatible with evidence that MDD and panic disorder subjects showed blunted thermic and adrenocorticotropin/cortisol responses to 5-HT$_{1A}$ receptor agonist administration (for review, see Drevets et al. 1999; Neumeister et al. 2004b).

The 5-HT$_{1A}$ receptor plays major roles in the neuroplasticity of serotonergic and other neurons (Azmitia et al. 1991; Brewton et al. 2001). During fetal development and subsequently during serotonin (5-HT) neuronal injury, stimulation of astrocyte and radial glial cell–based 5-HT$_{1A}$ receptors results in release of the trophic factor S100β, which promotes 5-HT neuronal arborization (Azmitia et al. 1991). Although it remains unclear whether the deficits in 5-HT$_{1A}$ receptor expression and glial cells constitute developmental or acquired abnormalities in mood disorders, it is noteworthy that reduced glial function during neurodevelopment conceivably could result in attenuated arborization of 5-HT neurons. Such a process could account for the widespread reductions of serotonin transporter (5-HTT) and postsynaptic 5-HT$_{1A}$ receptor expression seen in MDD (Bowen et al. 1989; Drevets et al. 1999; Mann et al. 2000; Parsey et al. 2002; Sargent et al. 2000) and the abnormal reduction in the area expressing 5-HT$_{1A}$ receptors in the dorsal raphe nucleus found in depressed persons who died by suicide (Arango et al. 2001). Notably, the persistently increased anxiety behaviors shown by 5-HT$_{1A}$ receptor knockout mice appear to result from deficient 5-HT$_{1A}$ receptor function on neuroplasticity during development (reviewed in Neumeister et al. 2004b).

CONCLUSION

The results of studies using neuroimaging, lesion analysis, and postmortem techniques converge to indicate that the pathophysiology of affective disorders involves dysfunction within PFC, limbic, striatal, and brainstem systems that modulate emotional behavior. Antidepressant and mood-stabilizing therapies may compensate for this dysfunction by attenuating the pathological limbic activity that mediates depressive signs and symptoms (Drevets et al. 2002a, 2002b) and by increasing transcription of neurotrophic factors that exert neuroplastic effects in pathways that modulate emotional expression (Manji et al. 2001).

REFERENCES

Abercrombie HC, Schaefer SM, Larson CL, et al: Metabolic rate in the right amygdala predicts negative affect in depressed patients. Neuroreport 9: 3301–3307, 1998

Alonso G: Prolonged corticosterone treatment of adult rats inhibits the proliferation of oligodendrocyte progenitors present throughout white and gray matter regions of the brain. Glia 31:219–231, 2000

Altshuler LL, Bartzokis G, Thomas G, et al: Amygdala enlargement in bipolar disorder and hippocampal reduction in schizophrenia: an MRI study demonstrating neuroanatomic specificity. Arch Gen Psychiatry 55:663–664, 1998

Amaral DG, Insausti R: Retrograde transport of D-[^{3}H]-aspartate injected into the monkey amygdaloid complex. Exp Brain Res 88:375–388, 1992

American Psychiatric Association: Diagnostic and Statistical Manual of Mental Disorders, 4th Edition, Text Revision. Washington, DC, American Psychiatric Association, 2000

Arango V, Underwood MD, Boldrini M, et al: Serotonin 1A receptors, serotonin transporter binding and serotonin transporter mRNA expression in the brainstem of depressed suicide victims. Neuropsychopharmacology 25:892–903, 2001

Ashtari M, Greenwald BS, Kramer-Ginsberg E, et al: Hippocampal/amygdala volumes in geriatric depression. Psychol Med 29:629–638, 1999

Axelson D, Doraiswamy PM, McDonald WM, et al: Hypercortisolemia and amygdala hippocampal changes in depression. Psychiatry Res 47:167–173, 1993

Azmitia EC, Whitaker-Azmitia PM: Awakening the sleeping giant: anatomy and plasticity of the brain serotonergic system. J Clin Psychiatry 52(suppl): 4–16, 1991

Bain EE, Nugent AC, Carson RE, et al: Decreased 5-HT1A receptor binding in bipolar depression. Biol Psychiatry 55:178S, 2004

Baumann B, Danos P, Krell D, et al: Reduced volume of limbic system-affiliated basal ganglia in mood disorders: preliminary data from a postmortem study. J Neuropsychiatry Clin Neurosci 11:71–78, 1999

Baxter LR, Schwartz JM, Phelps ME, et al: Reduction of prefrontal cortex glucose metabolism common to three types of depression. Arch Gen Psychiatry 46:243–250, 1989

Bell KA, Kupfer DJ, Drevets WC: Decreased glucose metabolism in the dorsomedial prefrontal cortex in depression. Biol Psychiatry 45:118S, 1999

Bench CJ, Friston KJ, Brown RG, et al: The anatomy of melancholia: focal abnormalities of cerebral blood flow in major depression. Psychol Med 22:607–615, 1992

Bench CJ, Friston KJ, Brown RG, et al: Regional cerebral blood flow in depression measured by positron emission tomography: the relationship with clinical dimensions. Psychol Med 23:579–590, 1993

Benes FM, Vincent SL, Todtenkopf M: The density of pyramidal and nonpyramidal neurons in anterior cingulate cortex of schizophrenic and bipolar subjects. Biol Psychiatry 50:395–406, 2001

Blumberg HP, Kaufman J, Martin A, et al: Amygdala and hippocampal volumes in adolescents and adults with bipolar disorder. Arch Gen Psychiatry. 60:1201–1208, 2003

Botteron KN, Raichle ME, Heath AC, et al: An epidemiological twin study of prefrontal neuromorphometry in early onset depression. Biol Psychiatry 45:59S, 1999

Botteron KN, Raichle ME, Drevets WC, et al: Volumetric reduction in left subgenual prefrontal cortex in early onset depression. Biol Psychiatry 51:342–344, 2002

Bowen DM, Najlerahim A, Procter AW, et al: Circumscribed changes of the cerebral cortex in neuropsychiatric disorders of later life. Proc Natl Acad Sci U S A 86:9504–9508, 1989

Bowley MP, Drevets WC, Öngür D, et al: Low glial numbers in the amygdala in mood disorders. Biol Psychiatry 52:404–412, 2002

Brambilla P, Harenski K, Nicoletti M, et al: MRI investigation of temporal lobe structures in bipolar patients. J Psychiatr Res 37:287–295, 2003

Brambilla P, Nicoletti M, Sassi RB, et al: Corpus callosum signal intensity in patients with bipolar and unipolar disorder. J Neurol Neurosurg Psychiatry 75:221–225, 2004

Bremner JD, Narayan M, Anderson ER, et al: Hippocampal volume reduction in major depression. Am J Psychiatry 157:115–118, 2000

Bremner JD, Vythilingham M, Vermetten E, et al: Reduced volume of orbitofrontal cortex in major depression. Biol Psychiatry 51:273–279, 2002

Brewton LS, Haddad L, Azmitia EC: Colchicine-induced cytoskeletal collapse and apoptosis in N-18 neuroblastoma cultures is rapidly reversed by applied S-100beta. Brain Res 912:9–16, 2001

Brody AL, Saxena S, Stoessel P, et al: Regional brain metabolic changes in patients with major depression treated with either paroxetine or interpersonal therapy: preliminary findings. Arch Gen Psychiatry 58:631–640, 2001

Buchsbaum MS, Wu J, Siegel BV, et al: Effect of sertraline on regional metabolic rate in patients with affective disorder. Biol Psychiatry 41:15–22, 1997

Carney RM, Freedland KE, Rich MW, et al: Ventricular tachycardia and psychiatric depression in patients with coronary artery disease. Am J Med 95:23–28, 1993

Charney DS, Drevets WC: The neurobiological basis of anxiety disorders, in Psychopharmacology: The Fifth Generation of Progress. Edited by Davis K, Charney DS, Coyle J, et al. New York, Lippincott Williams & Wilkins, 2002, pp 901–930

Cheng JD, de Vellis J: Oligodendrocytes as glucocorticoids target cells: functional analysis of the glycerol phosphate dehydrogenase gene. J Neurosci Res 59:436–445, 2000

Cotter D, Mackay D, Beasley C, et al: Reduced glial density and neuronal volume in major depressive disorder and schizophrenia in the anterior cingulate cortex. Schizophr Res 41:106, 2000

Cotter DR, Pariante CM, Everall IP: Glial cell abnormalities in major psychiatric disorders: the evidence and implications. Brain Res Bull 55:585–595, 2001a

Cotter DR, Mackay D, Landau S, et al: Reduced glial cell density and neuronal size in the anterior cingulate cortex in major depressive disorder. Arch Gen Psychiatry 58:545–553, 2001b

Cotter D, Mackay D, Chana G, et al: Reduced neuronal size and glial cell density in area 9 of the dorsolateral prefrontal cortex in subjects with major depressive disorder. Cereb Cortex 12:386–394, 2002

Damasio AR: Descartes' Error: Emotion, Reason, and the Human Brain. New York, Grosset/Putnam, 1995

Damasio A, Grabowski TJ, Bechara A, et al: Subcortical and cortical brain activity during the feeling of self-generated emotions. Nat Neurosci 3:1049–1056, 2000

D'Amelio F, Eng LF, Gibbs MA: Glutamine synthetase immunoreactivity present in oligodendroglia of various regions of the central nervous system. Glia 3:335–341, 1990

DelBello MP, Zimmerman ME, Mills NP, et al: Magnetic resonance imaging analysis of amygdala and other subcortical brain regions in adolescents with bipolar disorder. Bipolar Disord 6:43–52, 2004

Dewar D, Underhill SM, Goldberg MP: Oligodendrocytes and ischemic brain injury. J Cereb Blood Flow Metab 23:263–274, 2003

Dickstein DP, Treland JE, Snow J, et al: Neuropsychological performance in pediatric bipolar disorder. Biol Psychiatry 55:32–39, 2004

Dioro D, Viau V, Meaney MJ: The role of the medial prefrontal cortex (cingulate gyrus) in the regulation of hypothalamic-pituitary-adrenal responses to stress. J Neurosci 13:3839–3847, 1993

Drevets WC: Prefrontal cortical-amygdalar metabolism in major depression. Ann N Y Acad Sci 877:614–637, 1999

Drevets WC: Neuroimaging and neuropathological studies of depression: implications for the cognitive emotional manifestations of mood disorders. Curr Opin Neurobiol 11:240–249, 2001

Drevets WC: Neuroimaging abnormalities in the amygdala in mood disorders. Ann N Y Acad Sci 985:420–444, 2003

Drevets WC, Todd RD: Depression, mania and related disorders, in Adult Psychiatry, 2nd Edition. Edited by Guze SB. St. Louis, MO, Mosby (in press)

Drevets WC, Videen TO, Price JL, et al: A functional anatomical study of unipolar depression. J Neurosci 12:3628–3641, 1992

Drevets WC, Spitznagel E, Raichle ME: Functional anatomical differences between major depressive subtypes. J Cereb Blood Flow Metab 15:S93, 1995a

Drevets WC, Simpson JR, Raichle ME: Regional blood flow changes in response to phobic anxiety and habituation. J Cereb Blood Flow Metab 15:S856, 1995b

Drevets WC, Price JL, Simpson JR, et al: Subgenual prefrontal cortex abnormalities in mood disorders. Nature 386:824–827, 1997

Drevets WC, Öngür D, Price JL: Neuroimaging abnormalities in the subgenual prefrontal cortex: implications for pathophysiology of familial mood disorders. Mol Psychiatry 3:220–226, 1998

Drevets WC, Frank E, Price JC, et al: PET imaging of serotonin 1A receptor binding in depression. Biol Psychiatry 46:1375–1387, 1999

Drevets WC, Bogers W, Raichle ME: Functional anatomical correlates of antidepressant drug treatment assessed using PET measures of regional glucose metabolism. Eur Neuropsychopharmacol 12:527–544, 2002a

Drevets WC, Thase M, Bogers W, et al: Glucose metabolic correlates of depression severity and antidepressant treatment response. Biol Psychiatry 51:176S, 2002b

Drevets WC, Price JL, Bardgett ME, et al: Glucose metabolism in the amygdala in depression: relationship to diagnostic subtype and stressed plasma cortisol levels. Pharmacol Biochem Behav 71:431–447, 2002c

Drevets WC, Gadde K, Krishnan R: Neuroimaging studies of depression, in The Neurobiological Foundation of Mental Illness, 2nd Edition. Edited by Charney DS, Nestler EJ, Bunney BJ. New York, Oxford University Press, 2004a, pp 461–490

Drevets WC, Sills R, Nugent A, et al: Volumetric assessment of the amygdala in mood disorders using high resolution 3T MRI. Biol Psychiatry 55:182S, 2004b

Dupont RM, Jernigan TL, Heindel W, et al: Magnetic resonance imaging and mood disorders: localization of white matter and other subcortical abnormalities. Arch Gen Psychiatry 52:747–755, 1995

Eastwood SL, Harrison PJ: Hippocampal synaptic pathology in schizophrenia, bipolar disorder, and major depression: a study of complexin mRNAs. Mol Psychiatry 5:425–432, 2000

Eastwood SL, Harrison PJ: Synaptic pathology in the anterior cingulate cortex in schizophrenia and mood disorders: a review and a Western blot study of synaptophysin, GAP 43, and the complexins. Brain Res Bull 55:569–578, 2001

Escalona PR, McDonald WM, Doraiswamy PM, et al: Reduction of cerebellar volume in major depression: a controlled MRI study. Depression 1:156–158, 1993

Frodl T, Meisenzahl E, Zetzsche T, et al: Enlargement of the amygdala in patients with a first episode of major depression. Biol Psychiatry 51:708–714, 2002

Frysztak RJ, Neafsey EJ: The effect of medial frontal cortex lesions on cardiovascular conditioned emotional responses in the rat. Brain Res 643:181–193, 1994

Garcia R, Vouimba R-M, Baudry M, et al: The amygdala modulates prefrontal cortex activity relative to conditioned fear. Nature 402:294–296, 1999

George MS, Ketter TA, Parekh PI, et al: Brain activity during transient sadness and happiness in healthy women. Am J Psychiatry 152:341–351, 1995

Graybiel AM: Neurotransmitters and neuromodulators in the basal ganglia. Trends Neurosci 13:244–254, 1990

Hamidi M, Drevets WC, Price JL: Glial reduction in the amygdala in major depressive disorder is due to oligodendrocytes. Biol Psychiatry 55:563–569, 2004

Hauser P, Altschuler LL, Berrettini W, et al: Temporal lobe measurement in primary affective disorder by magnetic resonance imaging. J Neuropsychiatry Clin Neurosci 1:128–134, 1989

Herman JP, Cullinan WE: Neurocircuitry of stress: central control of the hypothalamo-pituitary-adrenocortical axis. Trends Neurosci 20:78–84, 1997

Hirayasu Y, Shenton ME, Salisbury DF, et al: Subgenual cingulate cortex volume in first-episode psychosis. Am J Psychiatry 156:1091–1093, 1999

Honer WG, Falkai P, Chen C, et al: Synaptic and plasticity-associated proteins in anterior frontal cortex in severe mental illness. Neuroscience 91:1247–1255, 1999

Husain MM, McDonald WM, Doraiswamy PM, et al: A magnetic resonance imaging study of putamen nuclei in major depression. Psychiatry Res 40:95–99, 1991

Jackson ME, Moghaddam B: Amygdala regulation of nucleus accumbens dopamine output is governed by the prefrontal cortex. J Neurosci 21:676–681, 2001

Johnston-Wilson NL, Sims CD, Hofmann JP, et al: Disease-specific alterations in frontal cortex brain proteins in schizophrenia, bipolar disorder, and major depressive disorder: the Stanley Neuropathology Consortium. Mol Psychiatry 5:142–149, 2000

Ketter TA, Kimbrell TA, George MS, et al: Effects of mood and subtype on cerebral glucose metabolism in treatment-resistant bipolar disorder. Biol Psychiatry 49:97–109, 2001

Kimbrell TA, Ketter TA, George MS, et al: Regional cerebral glucose utilization in patients with a range of severities of unipolar depression. Biol Psychiatry 51:237–252, 2002

Krishnan KRR, Doraiswamy PM, Figiel GS, et al: Hippocampal abnormalities in depression. J Neuropsychiatry Clin Neurosci 3:387–391, 1991a

Krishnan KRR, Doraiswamy PM, Lurie SN, et al: Pituitary size in depression. J Clin Endocrinol Metab 72:256–259, 1991b

Krishnan KRR, McDonald WM, Escalona PR, et al: Magnetic resonance imaging of the caudate nuclei in depression: preliminary observations. Arch Gen Psychiatry 49:553–557, 1992

Krishnan KRR, McDonald WM, Doraiswamy PM, et al: Neuroanatomical substrates of depression in the elderly. Eur Arch Psychiatry Neurosci 243:41–46, 1993

Kuroda M, Price JL: Synaptic organization of projections from basal forebrain structures to the mediodorsal thalamic nucleus of the rat. J Comp Neurol 303: 513–533, 1991

Lai T, Payne ME, Byrum CE, et al: Reduction of orbital frontal cortex volume in geriatric depression. Biol Psychiatry 48:971–975, 2000

Lenze EJ, Sheline YI: Absence of striatal volume differences between depressed subjects with no comorbid medical illness and matched comparison subjects. Am J Psychiatry 156:1989–1991, 1999

Links JM, Zubieta JK, Meltzer CC, et al: Influence of spatially heterogeneous background activity on "hot object" quantitation in brain emission computed tomography. J Comput Assist Tomogr 20:680–687, 1996

Lopez JF, Chalmers DT, Little KY, et al: A.E. Bennett Research Award. Regulation of serotonin 1A, glucocorticoid, and mineralocorticoid receptor in rat and human hippocampus: implications for the neurobiology of depression. Biol Psychiatry 43:547–573, 1998

Ludwin SK: The function of perineuronal satellite oligodendrocytes: an immunohistochemical study. Neuropathol Appl Neurobiol 10:143–149, 1984

MacFall JR, Payne ME, Provenzale JE, et al: Medial orbital frontal lesions in late onset depression. Biol Psychiatry 49:803–806, 2001

MacQueen GM, Campbell S, McEwen BS, et al: Course of illness, hippocampal function, and hippocampal volume in major depression. Proc Natl Acad Sci U S A 100:1387–1392, 2003

Magistretti PJ, Pellerin L: Cellular mechanisms of brain imaging metabolism and their relevance to functional brain imaging. Philos Trans R Soc Lond B Biol Sci 354:1155–1163, 1999

Manji H, Drevets WC, Charney D: The cellular neurobiology of depression. Nat Med 7:541–547, 2001

Mann JJ, Huang YY, Underwood MD, et al: A serotonin transporter gene promoter polymorphism (5-HTTLPR) and prefrontal cortical binding in major depression and suicide. Arch Gen Psychiatry 57:729–738, 2000

Martinez P, Ronsaville D, Gold PW, et al: Morphometric abnormalities in adolescent offspring of depressed mothers. Soc Neurosci Abstr 32, 2002

Matsuda Y, Fujimura K: Responses of the medial prefrontal cortex to stimulation of the amygdala in the rat: a study with laminar field potential recording. Neurosci Res 23:281–288, 1995

Matute C, Sanchez-Gomez MV, Martinez-Millan L, et al: Glutamate receptor-mediated toxicity in optic nerve oligodendrocytes. PNAS 94:8830–8835, 1997

Mayberg HS, Starkstein SE, Sadzot B, et al: Selective hypometabolism in the inferior frontal lobe in depressed patients with Parkinson's disease. Ann Neurol 28:57–64, 1990

Mayberg HS, Starkstein SE, Morris PL, et al: Remote cortical hypometabolism following focal basal ganglia injury: relationship to secondary changes in mood. Neurology 41(suppl):266, 1991

Mayberg HS, Starkstein SE, Peyser CE, et al: Paralimbic frontal lobe hypometabolism in depression associated with Huntington's disease. Neurology 42:1791–1797, 1992

Mayberg HS, Lewis PJ, Reginald W, et al: Paralimbic hypoperfusion in unipolar depression. J Nucl Med 35:929–934, 1994

Mayberg HS, Brannan SK, Mahurin RK, et al: Cingulate function in depression: a potential predictor of treatment response. Neuroreport 8:1057–1061, 1997

Mayberg HS, Liotti M, Brannan SK, et al: Reciprocal limbic-cortical function and negative mood: converging PET findings in depression and normal sadness. Am J Psychiatry 156:675–682, 1999

Mazziotta JC, Phelps ME, Plummer D, et al: Quantitation in positron emission computed tomography, 5: physical-anatomical effects. J Comput Assist Tomogr 5:734–743, 1981

McDonald AJ: Neuronal localization of glutamate receptor subunits in the basolateral amygdala. Neuroreport 6:13–6, 1994

McEwen BS, Magarinos AM: Stress and hippocampal plasticity: implications for the pathophysiology of affective disorders. Hum Psychopharmacol 16:S7–S19, 2001

Mervaala E, Fohr J, Kononen M, et al: Quantitative MRI of the hippocampus and amygdala in severe depression. Psychol Med 30:117–125, 2000

Mogenson GJ, Brudzynski SM, Wu M, et al: From motivation to action: a review of dopaminergic regulation of limbic → nucleus accumbens → ventral pallidum → pedunculopontine nucleus circuitries involved in limbic-motor integration, in Limbic Motor Circuits and Neuropsychiatry. Edited by Kalivas PW, Barnes CD. London, England, CRC Press, 1993, pp 193–236

Morgan MA, LeDoux JE: Differential contribution of dorsal and ventral medial prefrontal cortex to the acquisition and extinction of conditioned fear in rats. Behav Neurosci 109:681–688, 1995

Neumeister A, Nugent AC, Waldeck T, et al: Behavioral and neural responses to tryptophan depletion in unmedicated remitted patients with major depressive disorder and controls. Arch Gen Psychiatry 61:765–773, 2004a

Neumeister A, Bain E, Nugent A, et al: Reduced serotonin type 1A receptor binding in panic disorder. J Neurosci 24:589–591, 2004b

Nofzinger EA, Nichols TE, Meltzer CC, et al: Changes in forebrain function from waking to REM-sleep in depression: preliminary analyses of [18F]FDG PET studies. Psychiatry Res 91:59–78, 1999

Noga JT, Vladar K, Torrey EF: A volumetric magnetic resonance imaging study of monozygotic twins discordant for bipolar disorder. Psychiatry Res 106:25–34, 2001

Nowak G, Ordway GA, Paul IA: Alterations in the N-methyl-D-aspartate (NMDA) receptor complex in the frontal cortex of suicide victims. Brain Res 675:157–164, 1995

Nugent AC, Wood S, Bain EE, et al: High resolution MRI neuromorphometric assessment of the hippocampal subiculum in mood disorders. Presented at the International Society for Magnetic Resonance in Medicine 12th Scientific Meeting, Kyoto, Japan, May 2004

Öngür D, Price JL: The organization of networks within the orbital and medial prefrontal cortex of rats, monkeys, and humans. Cereb Cortex 10:206–219, 2000

Öngür D, Drevets WC, Price JL: Glial reduction in the subgenual prefrontal cortex in mood disorders. Proc Natl Acad Sci U S A 95:13290–13295, 1998

Osuch EA, Ketter TA, Kimbrell TA, et al: Regional cerebral metabolism associated with anxiety symptoms in affective disorder patients. Biol Psychiatry 48:1020–1023, 2000

Oya H, Howard M, Kawasaki H, et al: Intracranial field potentials recorded from the human amygdala and frontal cortex: amplitude and phase responses to emotional stimuli. Soc Neurosci Abstr 645.6, 2001

Pantel J, Schroder J, Essig M, et al: Quantitative magnetic resonance imaging in geriatric depression and primary degenerative dementia. J Affect Disord 42:69–83, 1997

Pearlson GD, Barta PE, Powers RE, et al: Medial and superior temporal gyral volumes and cerebral asymmetry in schizophrenia versus bipolar disorder. Biol Psychiatry 41:1–14, 1997

Perez-Jaranay JM, Vives F: Electrophysiological study of the response of medial prefrontal cortex neurons to stimulation of the basolateral nucleus of the amygdala in the rat. Brain Res 564:97–101, 1991

Pizzagalli D, Pascual Marqui RD, Nitschke JB, et al: Anterior cingulate activity predicts degree of treatment response in major depression: evidence from brain electrical tomography analysis. Am J Psychiatry 158:405–415, 2001

Price JL, Carmichael ST, Drevets WC: Networks related to the orbital and medial prefrontal cortex: a substrate for emotional behavior? Prog Brain Res 107:523–536, 1996

Raichle ME: Circulatory and metabolic correlates of brain function in normal humans, in Handbook of Physiology: The Nervous System, V. Edited by Brookhart JM, Mountcastle VB. Baltimore, MD, American Physiological Society, 1987, pp 643–674

Rajkowska G, Miguel-Hidalgo JJ, Wei Jinrong, et al: Morphometric evidence for neuronal and glial prefrontal cell pathology in major depression. Biol Psychiatry 45:1085–1098, 1999

Rajkowska G, Halaris A, Selemon LD: Reductions in neuronal and glial density characterize the dorsolateral prefrontal cortex in bipolar disorder. Biol Psychiatry 49:741–752, 2001

Rainnie DG, Asprodini EK, Shinnick-Gallagher P: Excitatory transmission in the basolateral amygdala. J Neurophysiol 66:986–998, 1991

Rauch SL, Jenike MA, Alpert NM, et al: Regional cerebral blood flow measured during symptom provocation in obsessive-compulsive disorder using oxygen 15-labeled carbon dioxide and positron emission tomography. Arch Gen Psychiatry 51:62–70, 1994

Ring HA, Bench CJ, Trimble MR, et al: Depression in Parkinson's disease: a positron emission study. Br J Psychiatry 165:333–339, 1994

Rolls ET: A theory of emotion and consciousness, and its application to understanding the neural basis of emotion, in The Cognitive Neurosciences. Edited by Gazzaniga M. Cambridge, MA, MIT Press, 1995, pp 1091–1106

Rosenkranz JA, Grace AA: Cellular mechanisms of infralimbic and prelimbic prefrontal cortical inhibition and dopaminergic modulation of basolateral amygdala neurons in vivo. J Neurosci 22:324–337, 2002

Rosoklija G, Toomayan G, Ellis SP, et al: Structural abnormalities in subicular dendrites in subjects with schizophrenia and mood disorders. Arch Gen Psychiatry 57:349–356, 2000

Sargent PA, Kjaer KH, Bench CJ, et al: Brain serotonin 1A receptor binding measured by positron emission tomography with [11C]WAY-100635: effects of depression and antidepressant treatment. Arch Gen Psychiatry 57:174–180, 2000

Saxena S, Brody AL, Ho ML, et al: Differential cerebral metabolic changes with paroxetine treatment of obsessive-compulsive disorder vs major depression. Arch Gen Psychiatry 59:250–261, 2002

Schultz W: Dopamine neurons and their role in reward mechanisms. Curr Opin Neurobiol 7:191–197, 1997

Schneider F, Gur RE, Alavi A, et al: Mood effects on limbic blood flow correlate with emotion self-rating: a PET study with oxygen-15 labeled water. Psychiatry Res Neuroimaging 61:265–283, 1995

Shah SA, Doraiswamy PM, Husain MM, et al: Posterior fossa abnormalities in major depression: a controlled magnetic resonance imaging study. Acta Psychiatr Scand 85:474–479, 1992

Shah PJ, Ebmeier KP, Glabus MF, et al: Cortical grey matter reductions associated with treatment-resistant chronic unipolar depression. Controlled magnetic resonance imaging study. Br J Psychiatry 172:527–532, 1998

Sheline YI, Wang PW, Gado MH, et al: Hippocampal atrophy in recurrent major depression. Proc Natl Acad Sci U S A 93:3908–3913, 1996

Sheline YI, Gado MH, Price JL, Amygdala core nuclei volumes are decreased in recurrent major depression. Neuroreport 9:2023–2028, 1998

Sheline YI, Sanghavi M, Mintun MA, et al: Depression duration but not age predicts hippocampal volume loss in medically healthy women with recurrent major depression. J Neurosci 19:5034–5043, 1999

Shen J, Petersen KF, Behar KL, et al: Determination of the rate of the glutamate/glutamine cycle in the human brain by in vivo 13C NMR. Proc Natl Acad Sci U S A 96:8235–8240, 1999

Shulman RG, Rothman DL: Interpreting functional imaging studies in terms of neurotransmitter cycling. Proc Natl Acad Sci U S A 95:11993–11998, 1998

Sibson NR, Dhankhar A, Mason GF, et al: Stoichiometric coupling of brain glucose metabolism and glutamatergic neuronal activity. Proc Natl Acad Sci U S A 95:316–321, 1998

Siegle GJ, Steinhauer SR, Thase ME, et al: Can't shake that feeling: event-related fMRI assessment of sustained amygdala activity in response to emotional information in depressed individuals. Biol Psychiatry 51:693–707, 2002

Siegle GJ, Konecky RO, Thase ME, et al: Relationships between amygdala volume and activity during emotional information processing tasks in depressed and never-depressed individuals: an fMRI investigation. Ann N Y Acad Sci 985:481–484, 2003

Steffens DC, Byrum CE, McQuoid DR, et al: Hippocampal volume in geriatric depression. Biol Psychiatry 48:301–309, 2000

Strakowski SM, DelBello MP, Sax KW, et al: Brain magnetic resonance imaging of structural abnormalities in bipolar disorder. Arch Gen Psychiatry 56:254–260, 1999

Sullivan RM, Gratton A: Lateralized effects of medial prefrontal cortex lesions on neuroendocrine and autonomic stress responses in rats. J Neurosci 19:2834–2840, 1999

Swayze VW II, Andreasen NC, Alliger RJ, et al: Subcortical and temporal structures in affective disorder and schizophrenia: a magnetic resonance imaging study. Biol Psychiatry 31:221–240, 1992

Thomas KM, Drevets WC, Dahl RE, et al: Abnormal amygdala response to faces in anxious and depressed children. Arch Gen Psychiatry 58:1057–1063, 2001

Timms RJ: Cortical inhibition and facilitation of the defence reaction. J Physiol Lond 266:98P–99P, 1977

Uranova N, Orlovskaya D, Vikhreva O, et al: Electron microscopy of oligodendroglia in severe mental illness. Brain Res Bull 55:597–610, 2001

Uranova NA, Vostrikov VM, Orlovskaya DD, et al: Oligodendroglial density in the prefrontal cortex in schizophrenia and mood disorders: a study from the Stanley Neuropathology Consortium. Schizophr Res 67:269–275, 2004

Vakili K, Pillay SS, Lafer B, et al: Hippocampal volume in primary unipolar major depression: a magnetic resonance imaging study. Biol Psychiatry. 47:1087–1090, 2000

Veith RC, Lewis N, Linares OA, et al: Sympathetic nervous system activity in major depression. Arch Gen Psychiatry 51:411–422, 1994

Velasco JM, Fernandez de Molina A, Perez D: Suprarhinal cortex response to electrical stimulation of the lateral amygdala nucleus in the rat. Exp Brain Res 74:168–172, 1989

Videbech P, Ravnkilde B, Pedersen AR, et al: The Danish PET/depression project: PET findings in patients with major depression. Psychol Med 31:1147–1158, 2001

von Gunten A, Fox NC, Cipolotti L, et al: A volumetric study of hippocampus and amygdala in depressed patients with subjective memory problems. J Neuropsychiatry Clin Neurosci 12:493–498, 2000

Vyas A, Mitra R, Shankaranarayana Rao BS, et al: Chronic stress induces contrasting patterns of dendritic remodeling in hippocampal and amygdaloid neurons. J Neurosci 22:6810–6818, 2002

Vyas A, Bernal S, Chattarji S: Effects of chronic stress on dendritic arborization in the central and extended amygdala. Brain Res 965:290–294, 2003

Vythilingam M, Heim C, Newport J, et al: Childhood trauma associated with smaller hippocampal volume in women with major depression. Am J Psychiatry 159:2072–2080, 2002

Webster MJ, Knable MB, Johnston-Wilson N, et al: Immunohistochemical localization of phosphorylated glial fibrillary acidic protein in the prefrontal cortex and hippocampus from patients with schizophrenia, bipolar disorder, and depression. Brain Behav Immun 15:388–400, 2001

Wilson J, Kupfer DJ, Thase M, et al: Ventral striatal metabolism is increased in depression, and decreases with treatment. Biol Psychiatry 51:122S, 2002

Wooten GF, Collins RC: Metabolic effects of unilateral lesion of the substantia nigra. J Neurosci 1:285–291, 1981

Wu JC, Gillin JC, Buchsbaum MS, et al: Effect of sleep deprivation on brain metabolism of depressed patients. Am J Psychiatry 149:538–543, 1992

Yates WR, Jacoby CG, Andreasen NC: Cerebellar atrophy in schizophrenia and affective disorder. Am J Psychiatry. 144:465–467, 1987

CHAPTER 9

Neuroapoptosis During Synaptogenesis

A Final Common Path to Neurodevelopmental Disturbances

John W. Olney, M.D.

Seeking to establish the genetic and/or environmental causes of mental illness has been a major preoccupation of mental health researchers for many decades. There is a strong belief that pathological events early in life play an important role, but progress has been slow in identifying the responsible pathogenic agents and establishing critical vulnerable periods during which the developing nervous system is at heightened

Supported in part by National Institute on Aging grant AG 11355, National Institute on Drug Abuse grant DA 05072, National Eye Institute grant EY 08089, National Institute of Child Health and Human Development grant HD 37100 (Merit Award), and a National Alliance for Research on Schizophrenia and Depression 2000 Toulmin Distinguished Investigator Award.

risk. In this chapter, I describe recent findings, primarily from laboratory animal research, that provide new insights into a specific type of mechanism that almost certainly plays an important role in some, and perhaps in many, human neurodevelopmental disorders. At the heart of this mechanism is the biological fact that neurons in the developing brain are programmed to kill themselves if they fail to perform according to a predetermined schedule. Under normal circumstances, a small percentage of neurons are unsuccessful in making the appropriate connections and therefore commit suicide, a process referred to variously as "physiological cell death," "necrobiosis," or, in recent years, "apoptosis." It follows that if adverse environmental factors interfere and prevent developing neurons from performing according to schedule, neurons that would otherwise have developed normally and contributed to the functional capacity of the brain will be driven to commit suicide. Depending on the degree of interference, many or only a few neurons may be deleted from the developing brain, and the resulting neurobehavioral disturbances may be extensive and readily recognized or relatively slight and inconspicuous.

What is the evidence that environmentally induced developmental neuroapoptosis contributes to human mental disorders? The most incontrovertible evidence pertains to fetal alcohol syndrome (FAS), a human condition that is clearly induced by an environmental pathogen, ethanol, and that is known to result in a wide spectrum of neuropsychiatric disturbances, ranging from attention-deficit/hyperactivity disorder (ADHD) and learning disabilities diagnosed in childhood to a high incidence of adult onset psychiatric disorders, including major depressive illness and psychosis (Famy et al. 1998). Recently, we demonstrated in experimental animals that brief exposure to ethanol during the developmental period of synaptogenesis can cause millions of neurons to commit suicide (die by apoptosis) in the developing brain, and the mechanism of ethanol's apoptogenic action has been traced to a disruptive effect of ethanol on two important neurotransmitter systems—the N-methyl-D-aspartate (NMDA) glutamate excitatory system and the γ-aminobutyric acid–A (GABA$_A$) inhibitory system. The significance of these findings is not limited to ethanol and FAS; many other agents in the human environment can interfere in the same manner with these same neurotransmitter systems, and all such agents have the heretofore unsuspected potential to trigger neuroapoptosis during the synaptogenesis period of development.

It was a highly serendipitous path that led to these observations, a path that began with an inquiry into the relationship between excitotoxic and apoptotic cell death processes and the role of glutamate signaling in either or both of these processes. In the following section I summarize important new findings in this line of research and discuss their significance in relation to neurodevelopmental disorders.

THE APOPTOSIS VERSUS NECROSIS VERSUS EXCITOTOXICITY QUANDARY

In recent decades, neuroscientists have become increasingly interested in cell death mechanisms, especially apoptotic and excitotoxic mechanisms, and in the potential relevance of these mechanisms to human neurodegenerative diseases. More recently, researchers have begun addressing the question of whether excitotoxic cell death processes might be mediated by apoptotic mechanisms, or vice versa. Typically, consistent with the precedent set by Wyllie et al. (1980), neuroscientists have framed the issue in terms of an "apoptosis versus necrosis" dichotomy, and the reported findings have been contradictory and confusing. Excitotoxic cell death has been described as a necrotic process, as an apoptotic process, as sometimes one and sometimes the other depending on the intensity of the stimulus, or as a hybrid mixture of both processes on a continuum.

DISTINGUISHING BETWEEN EXCITOTOXIC AND APOPTOTIC NEURODEGENERATION

Both excitotoxic and apoptotic neurodegeneration are phenomena that were originally defined in terms of their ultrastructural characteristics. Therefore, in our initial attempt to clarify the relationship between these two phenomena, we performed a side-by-side ultrastructural comparison of a prototypic in vivo excitotoxic process (glutamate-induced degeneration of neurons in the infant rat hypothalamus) and a prototypic in vivo apoptotic process, physiological (programmed) cell death (PCD), the natural process by which biologically redundant or unsuccessful neurons are deleted from the developing central nervous system (CNS). In this study (Ishimaru et al. 1999), we demonstrated by electron microscopy that the sequence and types of changes that characterize prototypic apoptotic cell death are strikingly different from the sequence and types of changes that characterize prototypic excitotoxic cell death. In other studies (Olney and Ishimaru 1999), we have examined several additional cell death processes triggered by an excitotoxic mechanism and have determined that although excitotoxic cell death has several different ways of manifesting, none of these ways entails ultrastructural changes resembling prototypic apoptosis (PCD). Thus, by ultrastructural criteria, excitotoxic and apoptotic cell death processes can readily be distinguished from each other. In our analysis, we have given no consideration to the word "necrosis" because we believe that it is a misnomer that lends confusion rather than clarity to the quest for an understanding of cell death processes. This point of view is discussed in greater detail in a review article (Dikranian et al. 2001).

MECHANISMS OF CELL DEATH IN HYPOXIA/ISCHEMIA AND HEAD TRAUMA

Our results prompted us to undertake additional studies aimed at determining whether other examples of excitotoxic neurodegeneration in the in vivo mammalian brain could be distinguished from apoptosis, using PCD as a reference standard for recognizing apoptosis. One example we studied was hypoxia/ischemia in the developing rodent brain and retina. In this study (Olney et al. 2000), we found that the primary response to hypoxia/ischemia is excitotoxic neurodegeneration, and this is followed by a delayed apoptotic response whereby neurons, deafferented by the primary wave of excitotoxic cell loss, committed suicide. We also studied concussive head trauma in infant rats (Bittigau et al. 1999; Ikonomidou et al. 1996; Pohl et al. 1999) and found that head trauma triggers in the infant rat brain both an excitotoxic and an apoptotic cell death process and that these two cell death processes can be distinguished quite readily by ultrastructural and several other criteria, the most interesting of which was their response to treatment. We administered drugs that block NMDA glutamate receptors and found that these drugs protected against the excitotoxic cell death process (Ikonomidou et al. 1996) and, instead of protecting, caused a worsening of the apoptotic cell death process (Pohl et al. 1999).

Interestingly, quantitative assessment of the number of neurons killed at the impact site by an excitotoxic mechanism compared with the number killed at numerous distant sites by an apoptotic mechanism revealed that the magnitude of the apoptotic lesion (collectively) was considerably greater than that of the excitotoxic lesion (Bittigau et al. 1998). Treatment of pediatric head trauma with an NMDA antagonist drug would therefore be contraindicated because it would be expected to rescue a small number of neurons at the risk of killing a much larger number.

POTENTIAL OF SELECTED AGENTS TO INDUCE APOPTOSIS IN THE DEVELOPING RAT BRAIN

NMDA Antagonists

These findings raised an interesting question: because NMDA antagonists promote the apoptotic neurodegenerative process induced in the immature brain by head trauma, is it possible that they might also promote the spontaneous apoptotic neurodegenerative process that occurs naturally (independent of head trauma) in the normal developing brain? We found that, indeed, MK801 and several other NMDA antagonists, both competitive and noncompetitive, when administered to 7-day-old infant rats, triggered a massive wave of apoptotic neurodegeneration affecting many neurons in several major regions of the developing brain (Ikonomidou et al. 1999).

GABAmimetics and Sodium Channel Blockers

Evidence that blockade of NMDA receptors during synaptogenesis triggers apoptotic neurodegeneration suggested the possibility that interference in other neurotransmitter processes during synaptogenesis might also trigger apoptotic neurodegeneration. To explore this possibility, we administered numerous agents that interact selectively with one or another transmitter receptor system and obtained largely negative results, with the major exception that a robust apoptotic response was triggered by agents (benzodiazepines and barbiturates) that mimic or potentiate the action of GABA at $GABA_A$ receptors (Ikonomidou et al. 2000b). In addition, we observed a similar apoptotic response following administration of certain anticonvulsant agents (e.g., phenytoin and valproate) that are not considered GABAmimetics but rather suppress neuronal activity by blocking voltage-gated sodium ion channels (Bittigau et al. 2002; Dikranian et al. 2000; Ikonomidou et al. 2000a).

Ethanol

We also evaluated ethanol, which reportedly has both NMDA antagonist (Hoffman et al. 1989; Lovinger et al. 1989) and GABAmimetic (Harris et al. 1995) properties, and found (Ikonomidou et al. 2000b) that it triggers a neurodegenerative response that is even more robust than the response to MK801 or GABAmimetics. The apoptotic nature of the degenerative response was confirmed by electron microscopy (for a detailed ultrastructural exposition, see Dikranian et al. 2001) and is *Bax* dependent (Olney et al. 2001; Young et al. 2003) and involves activation of caspase-3 (Olney et al. 2002b), which are characteristic features of apoptotic neurodegeneration. We studied both rats (Ikonomidou et al. 2000b) and mice (Olney et al. 2002a) and found that either species shows a robust apoptotic neurodegenerative response to ethanol. The pattern of neurodegeneration induced in the 7-day-old mouse brain by ethanol is illustrated in silver-stained sections (DeOlmos and Ingram 1971) in Figure 9–1 and by activated caspase-3 immunocytochemistry in Figures 9–2 and 9–3. The window of vulnerability to ethanol-induced apoptosis in the rodent forebrain was found to be the same as the apoptosis induced by NMDA antagonists and GABAmimetics; it coincides with the period of synaptogenesis, also known as the brain growth spurt period. This period in rats and mice is largely confined to the postnatal period; it begins a day or two before birth (perhaps earlier for caudal portions of the CNS) and terminates at approximately 14 days after birth, whereas in the human it spans the last 3 months of pregnancy and extends into the first several years postnatally (Dobbing and Sands 1979). An important feature of these findings is that it requires only a single ethanol intoxication episode to cause many millions of neurons to commit suicide in the developing brain. In the most severely affected brain regions, the magnitude of cell loss following a high dose of ethanol (5 g/kg subcutaneously) is in the range of 45%–68% (Olney et al. 2002a; Figures 9–4 and 9–5).

IMPLICATIONS OF ETHANOL FINDINGS FOR FETAL ALCOHOL SYNDROME

Intrauterine exposure of the human fetus to ethanol causes a dysmorphogenic neuropathological syndrome (Clarren et al. 1978; Jones and Smith 1973; Jones et al. 1973; Swayze et al. 1997), including craniofacial malformations and a reduced brain mass, which is associated with a variety of neurobehavioral disturbances ranging from ADHD and learning disabilities in childhood (Streissguth and O'Malley 2000) to major depressive and psychotic disorders in adulthood (Famy et al. 1998). Although the distinctive multifaceted clinical picture, as originally described (Jones and Smith 1975), has come to be known as *fetal alcohol syndrome*, it is now recognized that the fetotoxic effects of ethanol can manifest as a partial syndrome composed largely of neurobehavioral disturbances ranging from mild to severe and unaccompanied by craniofacial dysmorphogenesis. Alcohol-related neurodevelopmental disorder (ARND) is a term

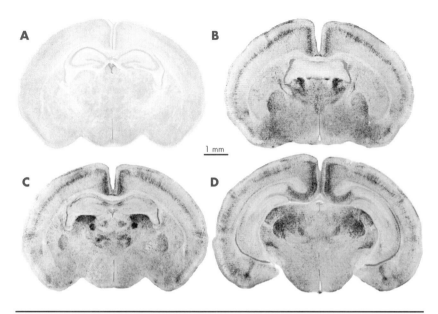

FIGURE 9–1.   Pattern of ethanol-induced apoptotic neurodegeneration at differ-ent rostrocaudal levels of the brain as revealed by silver staining.

These histological sections are from the 8-day-old C57BL/6 mouse brain 24 hours following subcutaneous treatment with saline (*A*) or ethanol (*B–D*). All sections are stained by the DeOlmos cupric silver method (DeOlmos and Ingram 1971), which causes neurons that are degenerating to be impregnated with silver. The photographs document that ethanol has triggered a robust neurodegenerative reaction throughout many regions of the mouse forebrain (each black speck is a degenerating neuron or fragment thereof), whereas saline has left the brain show-ing only a sparse pattern of apoptotic degeneration attributable to physiological cell death that occurs normally in the developing brain. The dying cells in the saline control are barely visible at low magnification because they are sparse in numbers, scattered in distribution, and often shrunken and fragmented. Note the remarkable bilateral symmetry of the ethanol-induced neurodegenerative reaction (*B–D*).

Source.   Adapted from Olney et al. 2002a.

recommended (Stratton et al. 1996) for referring to partial syndromes pri-marily affecting the CNS. Regardless of terminology, disruption of CNS development and consequent neurobehavioral disturbances are the most debilitating effects of ethanol on the developing human fetus.

Until recently, only limited success was achieved in developing suit-able animal models for studying FAS, and fundamental questions per-

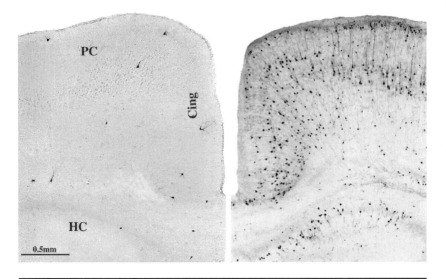

FIGURE 9–2.   Pattern of ethanol-induced caspase-3 activation in the rostral fore-brain.

These histological sections depict the parietal cortex (*PC*), cingulate cortex (*Cing*), and rostral hippocampus (*HC*) of the 7-day-old C57BL/6 mouse 8 hours after subcutaneous treatment with saline (*left*) or ethanol (*right*). Both sections have been stained immunocytochemically with antibodies to activated caspase-3. The saline control brain shows a pattern of caspase-3 activation that occurs normally in the 7-day-old mouse brain and is attributable to physiological cell death. These spontaneously degenerating neurons are more visible when stained by caspase-3 than by silver, because caspase activation occurs early while the neuron is still showing a well filled-out profile, and silver impregnation occurs later when the cell is condensed, shrunken, and/or fragmented. The pattern of caspase-3 activation closely resembles the pattern of silver staining shown in Figures 9–1B and 9–1C, but the density of caspase staining is not as great as the density of silver staining, because the silver stain marks all neurons that have degenerated over a 24-hour period, and caspase-3 immunocytochemistry marks only those neurons that are transiently undergoing caspase-3 activation at a given survival interval, in this case the 8-hour interval.

Source.   Adapted from Olney et al. 2002a.

taining to critical periods of vulnerability and to the nature of the neuropathological mechanisms remained unresolved. In the following paragraphs, I examine some of the unresolved issues and consider to what extent the new findings just described help clarify these fundamental issues.

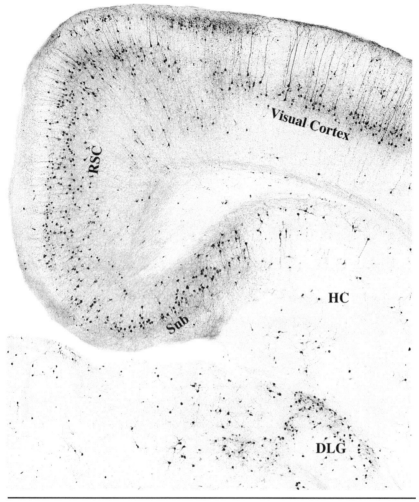

FIGURE 9–3. Brain section, stained immunocytochemically for activated (cleaved) caspase-3, from a 7-day-old mouse, 8 hours after a large dose of ethanol (5 g/kg subcutaneously).

This section is from the same rostrocaudal level as the silver-stained section in Figure 9–1D and displays the pattern of caspase-3 activation induced by ethanol in the visual cortex, retrosplenial cortex (*RSC*), subiculum (*Sub*), hippocampus (*HC*), and dorsolateral geniculate (*DLG*). Note that the caspase-3 activation pattern in these brain regions of the ethanol-treated pup is the same as the pattern of silver staining in these regions illustrated in Figure 9–1D. For illustrations documenting that very few neurons in this region of saline control brains show caspase-3 activation, see Olney et al. 2002a.

Source.   Adapted from Olney et al. 2002a.

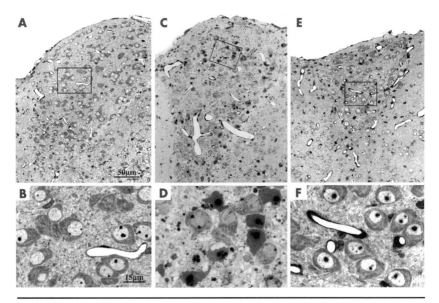

FIGURE 9–4. Ethanol-induced deletion of neurons from the anterodorsal nucleus of the thalamus (ADT).

These thin plastic sections depict the ADT nucleus of a 7-day-old mouse after saline treatment (*A, B*) or at 12 hours (*C, D*) or 72 hours (*E, F*) after ethanol treatment. The ADT neurons of the saline control brain (*A, B*) have a normal appearance, whereas at 12 hours after ethanol (*C, D*), many of them are grossly abnormal and display the typical features of apoptotic degeneration. At 12 hours, the ADT nucleus shows significant interstitial edema (*D*), but many of the individual neurons are condensed and shrunken, which causes the overall size of the nucleus to be slightly smaller than normal. In the interval between 12 and 72 hours, the dead neurons are debrided from the ADT nucleus by phagocytic cells, leaving the nucleus substantially reduced in neuronal mass, with a flattened contour by comparison with the saline control, which has a superior convexity that bulges out into the ventricle. Each of these brains was serially sectioned through the entire extent of the ADT nucleus and the section shown is from the nucleus at its maximum dimension. The cross section from the saline control has 155 normal neuronal profiles, whereas the section from the 72 hour ethanol treated animal has only 50. This represents a 68% reduction in neuronal mass. The ADT neurons 72 hours after ethanol, although reduced in number, have essentially a normal appearance.

Source.   Adapted from Olney et al. 2002a.

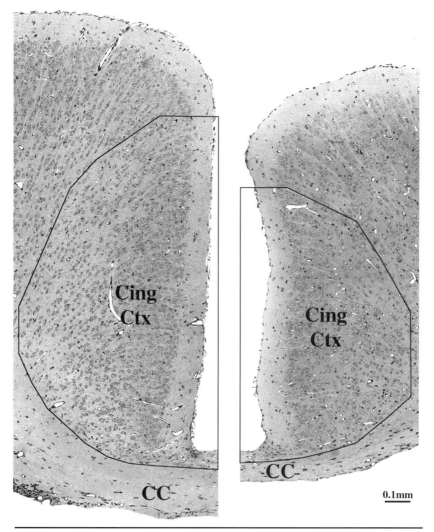

FIGURE 9–5. Impact of ethanol on the cingulate cortex and corpus callosum.

These panels depict the cingulate cortex and corpus callosum of the 10-day-old mouse brain 72 hours after treatment with saline (*left*) or ethanol (*right*). Both brain sections are shown at the same magnification and are cut from the same rostro-caudal level. Note the decreased cortical mass and also the decreased size of the corpus callosum (*CC*) of the ethanol-treated brain. Marked diminution of the corpus callosum has been reported as a typical neuropathological finding in fetal alcohol syndrome. The number of neuronal profiles within the demarcated area of the saline versus ethanol brain is 881 versus 488, which represents a 45% cell loss within the cingulate region.

Source. Adapted from Olney et al. 2002a.

Can the Apoptosis Process Explain the Neurobehavioral Disturbances Associated With Fetal Alcohol Exposure?

A point worth emphasizing is that ethanol-induced developmental neuroapoptosis can produce a wide variety of aberrant neurobehavioral outcomes. We have observed that, depending on whether exposure occurs during the early, middle, or late phase of synaptogenesis, ethanol triggers different patterns of neuronal deletion (Ikonomidou et al. 2000b), and it follows that each pattern has the potential to give rise to its own unique constellation of neurobehavioral disturbances. That this mechanism has the potential to contribute to a wide spectrum of neuropsychiatric disorders was documented by Famy et al. (1998), who found that 72% of FAS/ARND patients, after having experienced ADHD or learning disorders in childhood, required psychiatric care for adult-onset disturbances, including a 44% incidence of major depression and 40% incidence of psychosis.

An important goal of fetal alcohol research is to explain ethanol-induced learning disabilities, ranging from mild impairment to frank mental retardation. In the learning and memory literature, an "extended hippocampal circuit" has been described (Aggleton and Brown 1999) that, if disrupted, gives rise to learning and memory deficits. In addition to the hippocampus, this circuit is composed of the retrosplenial cortex, anterior thalamus, and mammillary complex. Our findings (Ikonomidou et al. 2000b; Olney et al. 2002a; Figures 9–1 through 9–5) document moderate loss of CA1 hippocampal neurons, severe loss of neurons in each of the other three regions composing the extended hippocampal circuit, dense degeneration of neurons in several layers and all divisions of the neocortex and limbic cortex, loss of a high percentage of the neurons that populate certain thalamic nuclei, and elimination of large numbers of neurons from the developing visual system, including the retina, lateral geniculate, superior colliculus, and visual cortex (Tenkova et al. 2003); the auditory system is also heavily affected at several levels, including the inferior colliculus, medial geniculate, and auditory cortex (J.W. Olney, unpublished data, 2005). Moreover, basal forebrain cholinergic neurons that pervasively innervate the neocortex, limbic cortex, and hippocampus are decimated. Given such extensive disruption of these many systems that play critical roles in learning, memory, sensory information processing, and cognitive function, it would be truly surprising if mental retardation were not a potential manifestation of this toxic syndrome.

In view of the Famy et al. (1998) finding that a high percentage of FAS/

ARND victims are found in adulthood to have adult-onset psychotic disorders, it is important to consider how psychotic outcomes might relate to early neuronal losses. A popular concept in psychosis research is that the thalamus normally filters information before relaying it on to the cerebral cortex, and when the thalamic filter is damaged, cerebrocortical neurons are flooded with, and begin responding chaotically to, unmodulated information. An additional relevant concept is that if certain neurons in the cerebral cortex that ordinarily maintain inhibitory tone at a cerebrocortical level are impaired or missing, this deficit will act in concert with the thalamic filter deficit to promote psychotic symptom formation. There is evidence that in patients with schizophrenia or manic psychosis, there is a deficit of inhibitory neurons in layer II of the cerebral cortex (Benes et al. 2001). In schizophrenia, neuroimaging evidence for structural deficits has also been reported in the thalamus (Andreason et al. 1994). Layer II cerebrocortical neurons and thalamic neurons are among those selectively deleted from the developing rodent brain by ethanol (see Figures 9–1 through 9–4). Thus, the rodent FAS model may provide valuable information regarding specific neuronal losses that correlate with psychotic outcomes. It will be important in future research to perform autopsies on human FAS/ARND victims who have a history of psychosis and determine whether there are deficits in these specific populations of neurons.

The glutamate dysfunction hypothesis of schizophrenia is one that has been gaining an increasing number of adherents in recent years. A version of this hypothesis that my coworkers and I have espoused (Olney 1989; Olney and Farber 1995) attributes the psychotic symptoms of schizophrenia to an NMDA receptor hypofunctional state that is instilled by some kind of pathogenic event in the in utero developing brain. When we first proposed this hypothesis, there was no known mechanism by which NMDA receptor hypofunction could be selectively instilled in the developing brain. However, the finding described herein that blockade of NMDA receptors during synaptogenesis causes widespread neuroapoptosis (Ikonomidou et al. 1999) provides the missing mechanism. Because the neuroapoptotic process entails blockade of NMDA receptors on neurons that are thereby suppressed and driven to commit suicide, the suicidal neurons that are being deleted from the brain are necessarily NMDA receptor-bearing neurons. Deletion of these neurons, together with their NMDA receptors, will result in a selective NMDA receptor hypofunctional state. Thus, treatment of immature animals with NMDA antagonist drugs may provide an interesting animal model for studying the neuroanatomical developmental substrates of schizophrenia.

Does Excessive Apoptosis, in a Stage Other Than Synaptogenesis, Play a Significant Role in Central Nervous System Dysmorphogenesis?

Disruption of neuronal migration resulting from ethanol's antagonist activity at NMDA glutamate receptors is a promising concept (Komuro and Rakic 1993) that requires more intensive investigation in the in vivo brain. If ethanol has a disruptive effect on migration, it remains to be determined whether this disruptive effect causes cells to commit suicide or to remain living but at an ectopic location. Dunty et al. (2001) reported that a single exposure of the developing rat embryo to ethanol during the period from gestation days 6.5–11 (a period comparable to the human first trimester) triggers apoptotic degeneration of certain progenitor cells destined to form craniofacial structures. These findings provide a likely explanation for the craniofacial malformations observed in FAS. These authors also described an increased rate of apoptosis in primitive cell populations destined to give rise to CNS structures and proposed that these findings may explain ethanol-induced CNS dysmorphogenic effects. In the final analysis, it seems likely that ethanol will be shown to exert an apoptogenic action not only during synaptogenesis but also at one or more earlier stages of neuronal ontogenesis. It is possible for this to be the case even if the main ethanol effect is primarily confined to the brain growth spurt period, because during this period many neurons are undergoing differentiation and migration at the same time that others are engaged in synaptogenesis.

By What Mechanism(s) Does Ethanol Ingestion Cause Developing Neurons to Undergo Apoptosis?

Is the dual mechanism we have proposed—blockade of NMDA receptors and hyperactivation of $GABA_A$ receptors—a valid explanation? If so, is it a full, or only a partial, explanation? On the basis of evidence described herein, I consider it likely that an NMDA antagonist and GABAmimetic mechanism contributes to ethanol's apoptogenic activity. However, at the present time this remains a hypothesis that is not proven. Moreover, it would not surprise me if one or more additional mechanisms are found to contribute to ethanol's apoptogenic activity. Once all relevant mechanisms are identified and confirmed, it will still be necessary to trace the sequence of steps by which these mechanisms cause the nerve cell to receive an internal signal to kill itself. Based on our finding that three different classes of agents (sodium channel blockers, NMDA antagonists, and GABAmimetics) all trigger neuroapoptosis, and in vitro evidence (Mennerick and Zorumski 2000; Xu et al. 2000) linking this effect to a reduction in neuronal activity, we have advanced the general proposal that an abnormal reduction in neuronal activity during the critical period of synaptogenesis is a condition to which the neuron is programmed to respond with an internal signal to kill itself. Hopefully, additional research will soon permit this global proposal to be replaced by a more specific operational explanation.

Once the Suicide Signal is Generated, What Are the Biochemical Pathways Through Which the Signal Is Executed?

In various apoptosis models, two major apoptotic pathways (extrinsic and intrinsic) have been described. The extrinsic pathway involves binding of cytokines to death receptors, activation of caspase-8, and cleavage and activation of effector caspases-3, -6, or -7. The intrinsic pathway is regulated by Bax and Bcl-XL, which are specialized proteins that have counterbalancing pro- and anti-apoptotic properties, respectively. After a death stimulus, the pro-apoptotic molecule Bax translocates to the mitochondrial outer membrane, where it has a disruptive influence that promotes increased membrane permeability and extra-mitochondrial leakage of cytochrome c, which triggers a sequence of processes culminating in the activation of caspase-3. In genetically normal mice, we found (Olney et al. 2002b) that ethanol triggers caspase-3 activation (Figures 9–2 and 9–3) in neurons throughout the various brain regions where ethanol-induced apoptotic neurodegeneration has been demonstrated by other methods, but it does not cause activation of caspase-8. This suggests involvement of the intrinsic, but not extrinsic, pathway in ethanol-induced apoptosis. Also implicating the intrinsic mitochondrial pathway is our recent finding (Young et al. 2003) that in the absence of the *Bax* gene (i.e., in homozygous *Bax* knockout mice) ethanol does not cause either caspase-3 activation or apoptotic cell death. Thus, it appears that ethanol-induced apoptotic neurodegeneration in the developing in vivo mammalian brain entails an action of *Bax* on mitochondrial membranes, causing abnormal release of cytochrome c and activation of the effector caspase-3, which is instrumental in executing a series of steps whereby the cell disassembles itself. Consistent with this interpretation is our ultrastructural observation (Dikranian et al. 2001) that one of the earliest morphological changes induced in neurons by ethanol is a distinctive alteration in mitochondria consisting of dissolution of the outer limiting membrane. Except for this evidence for early mitochondrial injury, all conspicuous early changes are in the nucleus and not the cytoplasm.

What Are the Threshold Conditions for Triggering Ethanol-Induced Apoptosis?

Although extrapolating from rodents to humans is an imperfect means of evaluating risk, it is a necessary and valuable first step. Therefore, we have begun examining the potential of ethanol and several other drugs or drug combinations to induce apoptotic neurodegeneration in the developing rodent brain and are attempting to identify threshold conditions that must be exceeded before neuroapoptosis will occur. Because apoptosis is the cell death process being evaluated, and because caspase-3 activation appears to be an invariable accompaniment of this cell death process and is easily detected at a cellular level, we have chosen to use activated caspase-3 immunocytochemistry as a marker for identifying and counting neurons that are undergoing apoptosis.

Previously we reported (Ikonomidou et al. 2000b) that for ethanol to induce a significant apoptotic response, the blood ethanol concentration would have to be elevated to 200 mg/dL and remain at that level for 4 hours. We now believe this estimate was substantially in error, the source of error being that the counts were performed on silver-stained sections 24 hours after ethanol administration, and at this time point sensitive neurons that underwent apoptosis in the early posttreatment interval had decomposed into small fragments that could not be identified (and counted) as dead neurons. Thus, after a low dose the most sensitive neurons in the brain were dying early and decomposing into an uncountable trace by 24 hours. We have now documented, using early caspase 3 activation as indicator of an apoptotic response, that transient blood ethanol elevations hovering in the 80 mg/dL range for approximately 60 minutes are a sufficient condition for triggering apoptotic neurodegeneration at a significantly higher rate than occurs in saline controls (Olney et al. 2002c).

Regardless whether the threshold in humans is higher or lower than in rodents, an important observation that is likely to have human relevance is that it only requires a single brief ethanol exposure to delete neurons from the developing CNS.

PUBLIC HEALTH IMPLICATIONS BEYOND
FETAL ALCOHOL SYNDROME

The recent findings reviewed herein constitute evidence for a new mechanism—brief suppression of neuronal activity during synaptogenesis—by which neurons on a large scale can be deleted from the developing brain. Fetal alcohol syndrome serves as witness that the developing human brain is exquisitely sensitive to this mechanism and that it requires only brief interference in synaptogenesis to trigger widespread apoptotic neurodegeneration. If only brief interference is required, the number of candidate factors that could cause such an interference may be quite large. Here I review those factors that have been identified thus far and discuss the potential impact this new mechanism may have on our thinking about the origins of neurodevelopmental psychiatric disorders.

Other Drugs of Abuse

Although ethanol is probably the most widely abused drug in modern society, and in human history, it is not the only drug of abuse that can damage the developing brain by its NMDA antagonist or GABA-mimetic properties. Other drugs that have one or the other of these properties and may be abused by pregnant mothers include phencyclidine (PCP, angel dust), ketamine (special K), nitrous oxide (laughing gas), benzodiazepines, and barbiturates.

Iatrogenic Neuroapoptosis

Iatrogenic exposure of the developing CNS to drugs that have apoptogenic properties is an issue that warrants careful attention. Most of the drugs used in obstetric and pediatric medicine to control seizure activity are either GABAmimetics or sodium channel blockers. Drugs from these two categories are often used in combination to achieve adequate control over seizures. We have demonstrated (Bittigau et al. 2002) that antiepileptic drugs in either of these categories trigger extensive neuroapoptosis in the developing rat brain, and combinations of antiepileptic drugs trigger much more severe neuroapoptosis than individual drugs. Also of concern is the fact that all drugs used in pediatric or obstetric anesthesia are either GABAmimetics or NMDA antagonists, and these drugs are typically used in combination to achieve an optimal level of general anesthesia. In a recent publication (Jevtovic-Todorovic et al. 2003), we described anesthetizing infant rats with specific drugs that are commonly used in pediatric anesthesia and observing that such anesthetic exposure causes widespread neuronal apoptosis in the developing brain and significant learning impairments that persist into adulthood.

AT THE END OF THE FETAL ALCOHOL SYNDROME/ALCOHOL-RELATED NEURODEVELOPMENTAL DISORDER RAINBOW: IS THERE A POT OF GOLD?

It is interesting to speculate that the potential significance of the findings discussed herein may transcend the context of fetal alcohol neurotoxicity, drug abuse, or iatrogenic brain damage. Glutamate and GABA are ubiquitous neurotransmitter/neurotrophic systems that have vitally important, but incompletely understood, roles in CNS development. There are many possible mechanisms by which these systems might be rendered dysfunctional during synaptogenesis. Moreover, if it requires only brief interference in synaptogenesis to trigger widespread apoptotic neurodegeneration, it is likely that there are neurotransmitter-unrelated factors yet to be discovered that can cause such a brief interference. For example, the synaptogenesis period coincides with the brain growth spurt period, a period during which the brain grows at a markedly accelerated rate because billions of neurons are all expanding their dendritic arbors to provide a larger surface area for receiving synaptic connections. Heavy metals are thought to disrupt protein synthesis that is required for the cytoskeletal expansion of the dendritic arbor. This could cause a developmental delay that might be interpreted by the neuron as a signal to commit suicide. Viral infections during pregnancy have been implicated as a causal factor in schizophrenia, but the mechanisms by which viruses might have a schizophrenogenic effect are not clear. Transient virus-induced neuronal dysfunction during synaptogenesis, serving as a trigger for neuroapoptosis, would be a possible mechanism. It is also possible that a disturbance at the genome level might be expressed as neuronal dysfunction during synaptogenesis, which would trigger neuroapoptosis as the operant mechanism, giving rise to a psychiatric disorder. Our findings suggest that whenever such interferences occur, they will silently drive neurons in large numbers to commit suicide and cause a child to be born with neurobehavioral disturbances of occult origin that may manifest either in childhood or adulthood, or both (Famy et al. 1998). Thus, we propose that this be considered a "final common pathway" type of mechanism which, regardless how it is activated, has considerable potential to disrupt brain development and give rise to a wide variety of neuropsychiatric disturbances.

CONCLUSION

In this chapter I have reviewed recent findings pertaining to a newly discovered mechanism—suppression of neuronal activity during syn- aptogenesis—that can cause large numbers of neurons to commit sui- cide and be permanently deleted from the developing brain. In humans, the period of synaptogenesis, also known as the brain growth spurt pe- riod, extends from mid-gestation to several years after birth. Three ma- jor categories of drugs—NMDA antagonists, sodium channel blockers, and GABAmimetics—that can cause neurons to commit suicide during synaptogenesis have been identified. Many of these agents are drugs of abuse to which the human fetal brain may be exposed during the third trimester by drug abusing mothers. Ethanol, the most widely abused drug in the world, triggers massive apoptotic neurodegeneration in the developing brain by interfering with both the NMDA and GABA$_A$ recep- tor systems. This likely accounts for the reduced brain mass and lifelong neurobehavioral disturbances associated with human FAS. Exposure of the immature brain to drugs in these three categories also occurs in the context of medical treatment, because many of these agents are used as sedatives, tranquilizers, anticonvulsants, or anesthetics in pediatric and / or obstetrical medicine. Because only brief interference in synaptogen- esis is required to trigger this neuroapoptosis response, and many fac- tors can potentially cause such brief interference, this final common pathway type of mechanism may contribute more frequently than we currently realize to psychiatric disorders of neurodevelopmental origin.

REFERENCES

Aggleton JP, Brown MW: Episodic memory, amnesia, and the hippocampal-an- terior thalamic axis. Behav Brain Sci 22: 425–489, 1999

Andreasen NC, Arndt S, Swayze V, et al: Thalamic abnormalities in schizophre- nia visualized through magnetic resonance image averaging. Science 266:294– 298, 1994

Benes FM, Vincent SL, Todtenkopf M: The density of pyramidal and nonpyra- midal neurons in anterior cingulate cortex of schizophrenic and bipolar sub- jects. Biol Psychiatry 50:395–406, 2001

Bittigau P, Pohl D, Sifrtinger M, et al: Modeling pediatric head trauma: mech- anisms of neurodegeneration and potential strategies for neuroprotection. Restor Neurol Neurosci 13:11–23, 1998

Bittigau P, Sifringer M, Pohl D, et al: Apoptotic neurodegeneration following trauma is markedly enhanced in the immature brain. Ann Neurol 45:724–735, 1999

Bittigau P, Sifringer M, Genz K, et al: Antiepileptic drugs and apoptotic neurodegeneration in the developing brain. Proc Nat Acad Sci U S A 99:15089–15094,
2002

Clarren SK, Alvord AC, Sumi SM, et al: Brain malformations related to prenatal
exposure to ethanol. J Pediatr 92:64–67, 1978

DeOlmos JS, Ingram WR: An improved cupric-silver method for impregnation
of axonal and terminal degeneration. Brain Res 33:523–529, 1971

Dikranian K, Tenkova T, Bittigau P, et al: Histological characterization of apoptotic neurodegeneration induced in the developing rat brain by rugs that
block sodium channels. Soc Neurosci Abstr 26:323, 2000

Dikranian K, Ishimaru MJ, Tenkova T, et al: Apoptosis in the in vivo mammalian forebrain. Neurobiol Dis 8:359–379, 2001

Dobbing J, Sands J: The brain growth spurt in various mammalian species. Early
Hum Dev 3:79–84, 1979

Dunty JR WC, Shao-yu C, Zucker RM, et al: Selective vulnerability of embryon-
ic cell populations to ethanol-induced apoptosis: implications for alcohol-
related birth defects and neurodevelopmental disorder. Alcohol Clin Exp Res
25:1523–1535, 2001

Famy C, Streissguth AP, Unis AS: Mental illness in adults with fetal alcohol syndrome or fetal alcohol effects. Am J Psychiatry 155:552–554, 1998

Harris RA, Proctor WR, McQuilkin SJ, et al: Ethanol increases $GABA_A$ responses
in cells stably transfected with receptor subunits. Alcohol Clin Exp Res 19:
226–232, 1995

Hoffman PL, Rabe CS, Moses F, et al: N-methyl-D-aspartate receptors and ethanol: inhibition of calcium flux and cyclic GMP production. J Neurochem 2:
1937–1940, 1989

Ikonomidou C, Qin Y, Labruyere J, et al: Prevention of trauma-induced neurodegeneration in infant rat brain. Pediatr Res 39:1020–1027, 1996

Ikonomidou C, Bosch F, Miksa M, et al: Blockade of glutamate receptors triggers
apoptotic neurodegeneration in the developing brain. Science 283:70–74,
1999

Ikonomidou C, Genz K, Engelbrechten S et al: Antiepileptic drugs which block
sodium channels cause neuronal apoptosis in the developing rat brain. Soc
Neurosci Abstr 26:323, 2000a

Ikonomidou C, Bittigau P, Ishimaru MJ, et al: Ethanol-induced apoptotic neurodegeneration and the fetal alcohol syndrome. Science 87:1056 1060, 2000b

Ishimaru MJ, Ikonomidou C, Tenkova TI, et al: Distinguishing excitotoxic from
apoptotic neurodegeneration in the developing rat brain. J Comp Neurol
408:461–476, 1999

Jevtovic-Todorovic V, Hartman RE, Izumi Y, et al: Early exposure to common
anesthetic agents causes widespread neurodegeneration in the developing
rat brain and persistent learning deficits. J Neurosci 23:876–882, 2003

Jones KL, Smith DW: Recognition of the fetal alcohol syndrome in early infancy.
Lancet 2:999–1001, 1973

Jones KL, Smith DW: The fetal alcohol syndrome. Teratology 12:1–10, 1975

Jones KL, Smith DW, Ulleland CN, et al: Pattern of malformation in offspring of chronic alcoholic mothers. Lancet 1:1267–1271, 1973

Komuro H, Rakic P: Modulation of neuronal migration by NMDA receptors. Science 260:95–97, 1993

Lovinger DM, White G, Weight FF: Ethanol inhibits NMDA-activated ion current in hippocampal neurons. Science 243:1721–1724, 1989

Mennerick S, Zorumski CF: Neural activity and survival in the developing nervous system. Mol Neurobiol 22:41–54, 2000

Olney JW: Excitatory amino acids and neuropsychiatric disorders. Biol Psychiatry 26:505–525, 1989

Olney JW, Farber NB: Glutamate receptor dysfunction and schizophrenia. Arch Gen Psychiatry 52:998–1007, 1995

Olney JW, Ishimaru MJ: Excitotoxic cell death, in Cell Death and Diseases of the Nervous System. Edited by Koliatsos VE, Ratan RR. Totowa, NJ, Humana Press, 1999, pp 197–219

Olney JW, Price MT, Labruyere J, et al: Perinatal hypoxia/ischemia kills neurons directly by excitotoxic necrosis and indirectly by deafferentation apoptosis. Soc Neurosci Abstr 26:1880, 2000

Olney JW, Tenkova T, Holtzman D, et al: Ethanol triggers widespread caspase-3 activation and apoptotic neurodegeneration in wild type but not Bax-deficient mice. Soc Neurosci Abstr 27:337, 2001

Olney JW, Tenkova T, Dikranian K, et al: Ethanol-induced apoptotic neurodegeneration in the developing C57BL/6 mouse brain. Dev Brain Res 133:115–126, 2002a

Olney JW, Tenkova T, Dikranian K, et al: Ethanol-induced caspase-3 activation in the in vivo developing mouse brain. Neurobiol Dis 9:205–219, 2002b

Olney JW, Tenkova T, Ikonomidou C, et al: Threshold conditions for triggering alcohol-induced apoptotic neurodegeneration in infant mouse brain. Program No 120.1., 2002 Abstract Viewer/Itinerary Planner. Washington, DC, Society for Neuroscience CD-ROM, 2002c

Pohl D, Bittigau P, Ishimaru MJ: Apoptotic cell death triggered by head injury in infant rats is potentiated by NMDA antagonists. Proc Nat Acad Sci U S A 96:2508–2513, 1999

Stratton K, Howe C, Battaglia F: Fetal Alcohol Syndrome: Diagnosis, Epidemiology, Prevention, and Treatment. Washington, DC, National Academy Press, 1996

Streissguth AP, O'Malley K: Neuropsychiatric implications and long-term consequences of fetal alcohol spectrum disorders. Semin Clin Neuropsychiatry 5:177–190, 2000

Swayze VW II, Johnson VP, Hanson JW, et al: Magnetic resonance imaging of brain anomalies in fetal alcohol syndrome. Pediatrics 99:232–240, 1997

Tenkova T, Young C, Dikranian K, et al: Ethanol-induced apoptosis during synaptogenesis. Invest Ophthalmol Vis Sci 44:2809–2817, 2003

Wyllie AH, Kerr JFR, Currie AR: Cell death: the significance of apoptosis. Int Rev Cytol 68:251–306, 1980

Xu W, Cormier R, Fu T, et al: Slow death of postnatal hippocampal neurons by GABA(A) receptor overactivation. J Neurosci 20:3147–3156, 2000

Young C, Klocke B, Tenkova T, et al: Ethanol-induced neuronal apoptosis in vivo requires BAX in the developing mouse brain. Cell Death Differ 10: 1148–1155, 2003

CHAPTER 10

Neurobiology, Neurogenesis, and the Pathology of Psychopathology

Charles F. Zorumski, M.D.

A major goal of psychiatric research is to understand the mechanisms involved in psychiatric disorders, with the hope that such understanding will result in improved diagnosis and more effective treatments. For this to happen, it is important for the field to incorporate advances in genetics and neurobiology. Examples of how this might occur are found in recent studies suggesting the importance of cell loss and neurogenesis in mood disorders. These studies represent a work in progress but provide an opportunity to consider how information from several scientific disciplines could shape the future of psychopathology.

BRAIN CELL LOSS IN PATIENTS WITH MOOD DISORDERS

The hippocampus, amygdala, and prefrontal cortex appear to be key components of neural systems underlying mood, and a growing literature indicates that patients with mood disorders exhibit structural changes in these regions. Many, but not all, neuroimaging studies report decreased hippocampal volumes in subjects with major depression and bipolar disorder (Harrison 2002). For example, Sheline et al. (1996, 1999) found that women with relatively long histories of depression had 10%–15% reductions in hippocampal volume but no change in cortical volume. Similarly, Bremner et al. (2000) reported 12%–19% decreases in hippocampal volumes in subjects with severe recurrent depression. The changes accounting for the hippocampal volume reductions are poorly understood but could reflect cell loss and synaptic rearrangement (Harrison 2002). An intriguing finding is that subjects with bipolar disorder have an approximately 40% decrease in nonpyramidal neurons in the CA2 hippocampal region with a similar trend in the CA3 region (Benes et al. 1998).

Individuals with familial major depression and bipolar disorder also exhibit volume reductions in the subgenual prefrontal cortex (Drevets et al. 1997). Öngür et al. (1998) found that subjects with these disorders have a predominant loss of glial cells in this region. Cotter et al. (2001b) reported decreased glial density and neuronal size in the supracallosal anterior cingulate cortex of subjects with major depressive disorder but no changes in subjects with bipolar disorder. Rajkowska et al. (1999; Rajkowska 2000) described a reduction in both neuronal and glial densities in the rostral orbitofrontal cortex with diminished glial density and neuronal size in the caudal orbitofrontal cortex and decreased size and density of glia and neurons in the dorsolateral prefrontal cortex in subjects with nonpsychotic major depression. In a study of bipolar subjects, Rajkowska et al. (2001) reported decreased neuronal and glial density in dorsolateral prefrontal cortex. Cotter et al. (2002) also observed reduced neuronal size and glial density in the dorsolateral prefrontal cortex in individuals with major depression.

Structural and cellular changes in other brain regions, including the amygdala, have received less attention. There is evidence for volume reduction in the amygdala of patients with mood disorders (Sheline et al. 1998), and one study found decreased glial density without neuronal loss in the left amygdala (Bowley et al. 2002).

These studies suggest that structural changes, including loss of glial cells and changes in both pyramidal and nonpyramidal neurons, occur in the brains of subjects with mood disorders. It is less clear whether the changes are restricted to specific illness subtypes or are specific to mood disorders. Some studies have observed effects in subjects with familial depression and bipolar disorder, but this finding is not consistent (Harrison 2002). Regarding illness specificity, it is notable that changes in the hippocampus and frontal cortex also occur in schizophrenia and posttraumatic stress disorder. There is also evidence for glial loss and decreased neuronal density in the prefrontal cortex of persons with schizophrenia, although the glial changes may be most prominent in those who also have depression (Cotter et al. 2001a, 2001b).

The timing of the brain changes remains uncertain but is important for determining contributing mechanisms. Cell loss at illness onset has different pathological implications than cell loss after a long duration of illness. Left hippocampal atrophy correlates with lifetime duration of depression (Sheline et al. 1996, 1999), multiple episodes of depression (MacQueen et al. 2003), and treatment resistance (Shah et al. 1998, 2002). However, Frodl et al. (2002) found that men with recent-onset depression have smaller hippocampal volumes at illness onset compared with healthy control subjects, with no differences observed in women. Similarly, Hiraysu et al. (1999) observed smaller left subgenual cingulate cortex volumes in first-episode subjects with psychotic mood disorders and a family history of mood disorder. Botteron et al. (2002) observed that the magnitude of changes in the left subgenual prefrontal cortex is similar in adolescent and middle-aged women with depression, suggesting that atrophy may be present early in the illness, perhaps antedating illness onset.

From the available data, it is premature to be confident of any specific pathological mechanisms. A popular hypothesis, particularly for changes that correlate with illness duration or severity, relates such changes to elevations in glucocorticoids (Sapolsky 2000). Some subjects with mood disorders exhibit altered cortisol secretion during depressed episodes, and studies in animals indicate that glucocorticoids can damage neurons, particularly in the hippocampus (Sapolsky 2000). However, evidence linking atrophy to altered cortisol secretion is lacking. Other possibilities include changes in neurotrophic factors or excitotoxicity.

An intriguing notion is that some changes may result from developmental abnormalities. The lack of gliosis in postmortem studies is consistent with this hypothesis, and Botteron et al.'s (2002) findings suggest that a developmental defect accounts for at least some changes in the prefrontal cortex. Individuals with smaller hippocampal volumes also appear to be at risk for pathological reactions to psychological trauma (Gilbertson et al. 2002), and smaller hippocampal volumes in depressed women may be associated with early childhood trauma (Vythilingham et al. 2002). These observations make it important to understand factors that affect cell survival during development. In many brain regions, more cells are generated than are required for mature function, with excess cells dying normally over the course of development. Neuro-trophic agents and neuronal activity help to determine which neurons survive (Mennerick and Zorumski 2000), but less is known about factors regulating glial survival.

Of potential importance are recent findings demonstrating that de-velopmental exposure to a variety of abused and therapeutic drugs has large effects on neuronal survival (Ikonomidou et al. 1999, 2000; Xu et al. 2000). Agents that augment inhibition (e.g., benzodiazepines, barbi-turates, anesthetics, and ethanol) or dampen excitation (e.g., ethanol, phencyclidine, and ketamine) greatly enhance neuronal death when ad-ministered for brief periods to rodents during synapse formation. Sim-ilar effects are observed with drugs that block voltage-activated sodium or calcium channels (Bittigau et al. 2002; Moulder et al. 2002), some of which are used clinically as anticonvulsants or mood stabilizers (e.g., phenytoin, carbamazepine). The neuronal loss caused by these drugs appears to result from dampened neuronal activity leading to apopto-sis. The untimely loss of neurons at critical stages of development in-fluences subsequent synaptic function and the ability of animals to learn as they mature to adolescence and adulthood (Jevtovic-Todorovic et al. 2003). Although these findings are most relevant to fetal alcohol syn-drome, it is not a great stretch to envision excessive developmental cell loss participating in the vulnerability to other neuropsychiatric syn-dromes. Indeed, individuals with fetal alcohol syndrome may have in-creased risk for major depression and psychosis in adulthood (Famy et al. 1998).

EFFECTS OF LITHIUM ON NEURONAL SURVIVAL

Given the effects just outlined, it is important to consider how treat-ments used in psychiatry affect cell survival. Moreover, given recent findings of deleterious effects of anticonvulsants and sedating drugs on the developing nervous system of animals, it is important to determine whether psychotropic medications administered early in life have ad-verse effects. The answers to these questions will require systematic in-vestigation into the longitudinal course of cellular and synaptic changes in psychiatric disorders. At present there is no convincing evidence that antidepressants, and antipsychotics, or lithium causes developmental cell loss. However, recent studies have provided interesting and, at times, surprising results. For example, it appears that chronic lithium treatment has neuroprotective effects against several forms of neurode-generation (Ikonomov and Manji 1999; Manji et al. 1999). Lithium also enhances the survival of developing neurons following growth factor withdrawal and supports the survival of cerebellar granule cells grown in culture. Cultured granule cells are very sensitive to trophic factor deprivation or withdrawal of depolarizing input and have served as a model for determining the role of trophic factors and activity during development.

The protective effects of lithium appear to involve pathways regulating apoptotic death. *Apoptosis* is a form of cell death characterized by cell shrinkage, nuclear dissolution, and intracellular inclusions and is normally a way that organisms rid themselves of unneeded cells (see Chapter 9: "Neuroapoptosis During Synaptogenesis"). Apoptosis, which occurs naturally during development and is regulated by neurotrophic factors and neuronal activity, is an active process using specific molecular programs. Among the agents that regulate apoptosis are members of the bcl-2 (B-cell lymphoma/leukemia-2) family of proteins. Some bcl-2 proteins promote death when activated, whereas others are protective. Bcl-2 is an anti-apoptotic protein that localizes to mitochondrial membranes, endoplasmic reticulum, and nuclear membranes and acts in part by regulating the release of cytochrome c from mitochondria. Cytochrome c leads to activation of cysteine-aspartate proteinases (caspases) that cleave intracellular proteins and cause cell death. Lithium appears to alter apoptosis by increasing bcl-2 expression (Manji et al. 1999, 2001). Lithium also decreases the pro-apoptotic protein p53 and inhibits GSK-3β (glycogen synthetase kinase), an enzyme involved in cell death pathways. Some effects of lithium, particularly those on bcl-2 and GSK-3β, are mimicked by valproate, another mood stabilizing agent.

ANTIDEPRESSANTS AND NEUROGENESIS

Evidence suggesting that antidepressants have neuroprotective effects is less certain. However, chronic stress in animals results in cell loss in specific brain regions. In a model of chronic social stress, tree shrews exhibit behavioral and endocrine changes reminiscent of depression in humans. Antidepressants reverse these effects (Fuchs and Flugge 2002). Similarly, the novel antidepressant tianeptine diminishes stress-induced volume changes in the hippocampus, suggesting neuroprotective actions (Czeh et al. 2001). Tianeptine also blocks inhibitory effects of stress on neurogenesis in the dentate gyrus, raising the question whether other antidepressants also affect neurogenesis. There is evidence in rats that chronic antidepressant treatment increases the number of new cells in the dentate gyrus (Malberg et al. 2000). Effective agents include fluoxetine, reboxetine, tranylcypromine, and electroconvulsive shock, which increase the number of proliferative cells by about 15%–40%. The effects of fluoxetine take weeks to occur, a time course akin to that required for antidepressant actions. Similarly, chronic lithium increases neurogenesis in the dentate gyrus of adult mice by about 25% (Chen et al. 2000). More recent studies using transgenic mice and treatments to inhibit neurogenesis provide strong evidence that some behavioral effects of antidepressants require neurogenesis in the dentate gyrus (Santarelli et al. 2003).

The effects on neurogenesis raise questions about how antidepressants exert their actions. Considerable evidence indicates that adult mammalian brains have two regions with high densities of neural progenitor cells—the subventricular zone of the lateral ventricle and the subgranular zone of the dentate gyrus. In the adult rodent dentate gyrus, about one new neuron is born per day per 2,000 existing neurons, reflecting 1,000–3,000 new dentate cells per day (Gage 2000). Neurogenesis decreases with advancing age, stress, and glucocorticoids and is augmented by exposure to enriched environments, voluntary exercise, caloric restriction, and learning (Gold and Gross 2002). Of potential importance for psychopathology is evidence that prenatal stress in rats diminishes proliferation in the dentate gyrus of adult offspring and dampens spatial learning and learning-induced neurogenesis (Lemaire et al. 2000).

The generation of new neurons and glia in the adult nervous system suggests that these cells could serve as a means to recover from illness or to enhance basal function. For this to happen, new cells must function in synaptic circuits. Although some estimates indicate that at least half of the new neurons die over a several week period (Dayer et al. 2003), some of the recently generated cells in the brains of adult animals develop properties of neurons, including the ability to fire action potentials and to form active synaptic connections with neighboring neurons (Mistry et al. 2002; Song et al. 2002a). Van Praag et al. (2002) studied this issue in some detail by labeling dividing cells in the brains of adult mice with a retroviral vector expressing green fluorescent protein (GFP). The GFP label allowed identification of recently generated cells in hippocampal slices prepared from the mice. By 4–8 weeks after generation, GFP-positive neurons joined the circuitry of the dentate and exhibited synaptic responses akin to preexisting neurons. Similarly, following ischemic damage to pyramidal neurons in the CA1 region of the rodent hippocampus, progenitor cells from the posterior periventricular region provided new neurons to the region, with the new neurons integrating into the CA1 circuitry and helping to diminish defects in learning (Nakatomi et al. 2002). The latter findings are of interest because CA1 has not previously been associated with neurogenesis or functional recovery following lesions.

These studies raise questions about why new neurons would be generated in certain circuits. On the basis of the importance of the hippocampus in memory, Kempermann (2002) suggested that new dentate neurons enable the hippocampus to process greater degrees of complexity. Support for this comes from studies in which voluntary exercise in rodents enhanced neurogenesis, spatial learning, and long-term potentiation in the dentate gyrus (Gould et al. 1999a; Van Praag et al. 1999). Long-term potentiation was not enhanced in the nearby CA1 region where new neurons did not form. *Long-term potentiation* is a synaptic mechanism thought to underlie certain forms of learning, particularly spatial learning in rodents. Similarly, treatments that reduce the number of new neurons in the dentate gyrus impair the ability of rats to learn a trace conditioning task, and recovery of neurogenesis is associated with the ability to learn the task (Shors et al. 2001).

NEUROGENESIS AND MOOD DISORDERS

For the neurogenesis story to be relevant to psychiatry, it is important to know whether neurogenesis occurs in the human nervous system and to determine whether changes in neuronal and glial numbers have effects similar to those observed in rodents. Again, evidence directly dealing with these issues is limited. However, neural progenitor cells can be isolated from the postmortem adult and infant human brain and, when grown in culture, develop neuronal and glial phenotypes (Palmer et al. 2001).

Present evidence indicates that diverse classes of psychotropic treatments, including, at a minimum, a serotonin uptake inhibitor (fluoxetine), a monoamine oxidase inhibitor (tranylcypromine), a norepinephrine uptake inhibitor (reboxetine), a novel antidepressant (tinaeptine), lithium, and electroconvulsive shock, enhance dentate neurogenesis. To the extent they have been tested, antipsychotics do not appear to share this property (Halim et al. 2004; Malberg et al. 2000; Wang et al. 2004). The findings with electroconvulsive shock are intriguing, given concerns about memory impairment with electroconvulsive therapy. To date, at least three studies have shown enhanced neurogenesis in the dentate gyrus of rodents following a series of electroconvulsive shocks that in some cases was specifically designed to mimic a course of electroconvulsive therapy (Madsen et al. 2000; Malberg et al. 2000; Scott et al. 2000).

These findings raise questions about the cognitive impairment that accompanies severe mood disorders and the ability of antidepressant treatments to improve mood symptoms and cognitive dysfunction. It is unknown whether antidepressants increase neurogenesis in the adult human nervous system. Indirectly, there is evidence that 4 weeks of lithium treatment increases N-acetyl aspartate levels in human gray matter (Moore et al. 2000a). N-Acetyl aspartate is an endogenous amino acid found in neurons that can be measured using magnetic resonance spectroscopy and is thought to provide an index of neuronal integrity (Manji et al. 2000). Additionally, 4 weeks of lithium increases total gray matter content in the human brain (Moore et al. 2000b). Other evidence indicates that subjects with bipolar disorder treated with lithium or valproate do not show glial loss in the amygdala compared with subjects not given lithium (Bowley et al. 2002). Finally, there is evidence that longer durations of untreated depression are associated with hippocampal volume loss but that no such relationship exists with time depressed while taking antidepressants (Sheline et al. 2003).

The effects of stress, glucocorticoids, and antidepressants on neurogenesis have prompted hypotheses about the biology of mood disorders. Jacobs et al. (2000) suggested that depressive disorders represent a defect arising from loss of neurons under the influence of stress and cortisol hypersecretion. By enhancing dentate neurogenesis, antidepressants reverse the process and stabilize mood. This hypothesis also suggests that more effective treatments for depression can be developed on the basis of the biology of cell loss and neurogenesis. Although speculative, one can imagine attempts to develop antidepressant and mood-stabilizing treatments based on inhibiting the effects of glucocorticoids, upregulating neurotrophic factors, or enhancing cell-survival pathways (Alonso et al. 2004). It is also possible that nonpharmacological psychiatric treatments affect neurogenesis. If psychotherapy is viewed as a form of learning, then, the rodent literature suggests, such treatment can also enhance neurogenesis. Furthermore, behavioral treatments that foster a healthy lifestyle, including regular exercise, an enriched environment, and a calorically restricted diet, may be beneficial for cognition and mood via enhanced neurogenesis. Thus, neurogenesis could represent a point of mechanistic convergence among psychopharmacological, electrical, psychotherapeutic, and behavioral treatments.

Among the many difficulties with this hypothesis is that there are primarily two regions in brain where neurogenesis is prominent in adults. However, both regions appear to be involved in the cell loss associated with mood disorders. Given the importance of the hippocampus and prefrontal cortex in information processing and mood, it is possible that having new cells in these regions may reverse a pathological process. Presently, most data deal with the dentate gyrus, and less is known about the prefrontal cortex and other brain regions. Gould et al. (1999b, 2001) reported evidence for neurogenesis in the primate prefrontal cortex, although these findings are debated (Rakic 2002). Other studies indicate that new neurons are generated in emotion processing circuits of the amygdala, piriform cortex, and inferior temporal cortex of primates (Bernier et al. 2002). It is also important to consider changes in glial cells in patients with mood disorders, because postmortem studies demonstrate a loss of these cells in regions of frontal cortex. Understanding factors that direct progenitor fate toward neurons or glia, as well as understanding the interaction between neurons and glia in the normal brain, will be important to make progress in this direction (Seri et al. 2001; Song et al. 2002b). Further knowledge about the importance of glia in information processing is likely to enhance interpretation of changes in brain function observed in neuroimaging studies (Schulman 2001).

CONCLUSION

The studies reviewed in this chapter suggest that structural changes occur in the brains of at least some patients with mood disorders. These structural changes result, at least in part, from a loss of both glia and neurons. Additionally, the evidence that psychiatric treatments increase neurogenesis in animals is reasonably strong. It is also becoming clear that antecedents for some adult psychiatric disorders lie in events that occur during childhood. Thus, studies demonstrating that exposure to a variety of abused and therapeutic drugs during key times in development greatly alters neuronal survival have implications for developmental models of psychopathology. Similarly, prenatal stress and early abuse are likely to affect neuronal and glial survival and neurogenesis. How the loss of both neurons and glia occurs and how this influences information processing is unclear but experimentally tractable. Furthermore, work on adult neurogenesis has implications for new directions in psychiatric therapeutics.

REFERENCES

Alonso R, Griebel G, Pavone G, et al: Blockade of CRF(1) or V(1b) receptors reverses stress-induced suppression of neurogenesis in a mouse model of depression. Mol Psychiatry 9:278–286, 2004

Benes FM, Kwok EW, Vincent SL, et al: A reduction of nonpyramidal cells in sector CA2 of schizophrenics and manic depressives. Biol Psychiatry 44:88–97, 1998

Bernier PJ, Bedard A, Vinet J, et al: Newly generated neurons in the amygdala and adjoining cortex of adult primates. Proc Natl Acad Sci U S A 99:11464–11469, 2002

Bittigau P, Sifringer M, Genz K, et al: Antiepileptic drugs and apoptotic neurodegeneration in the developing brain. Proc Natl Acad Sci U S A 99:15089–15094, 2002

Botteron KN, Raichle ME, Drevets WC, et al: Volumetric reduction in left subgenual prefrontal cortex in early onset depression. Biol Psychiatry 51:342–344, 2002

Bowley MP, Drevets WC, Ongur D, et al: Low glial numbers in the amygdala in major depressive disorder. Biol Psychiatry 52:404–412, 2002

Bremner JD, Narayan M, Anderson ER, et al: Hippocampal volume reduction in major depression. Am J Psychiatry 157:115–118, 2000

Chen G, Rajkowska G, Du F, et al: Enhancement of hippocampal neurogenesis by lithium. J Neurochem 75:1729–1734, 2000

Cotter D, Pariante CM, Everall IP: Glial cell abnormalities in major psychiatric disorders: the evidence and implications. Brain Res Bull 55:585–595, 2001a

Cotter D, Mackay D, Landau S, et al: Reduced glial cell density and neuronal size in the anterior cingulate cortex in major depressive disorder. Arch Gen Psychiatry 58:545–553, 2001b

Cotter D, Mackay D, Chana G, et al: Reduced neuronal size and glial cell density in area 9 of the dorsolateral prefrontal cortex in subjects with major depressive disorder. Cereb Cortex 12:386–394, 2002

Czeh B, Michaelis T, Watanabe T, et al: Stress-induced changes in cerebral metabolites, hippocampal volume, and cell proliferation are prevented by antidepressant treatment with tianeptine. Proc Natl Acad Sci U S A 98:12796–12801, 2001

Dayer AG, Ford AA, Cleaver KM, et al: Short-term and long-term survival of new neurons in the rat dentate gyrus. J Comp Neurol 460:563–572, 2003

Drevets WC, Price JL, Simpson JR, et al: Subgenual prefrontal cortex abnormalities in mood disorders. Nature 386:824–827, 1997

Famy C, Streissguth AP, Unis AS: Mental illness in adults with fetal alcohol syndrome or fetal alcohol effects. Am J Psychiatry 155:552–554, 1998

Frodl T, Meisenzahl EM, Zetzsche T, et al: Hippocampal changes in patients with a first episode of major depression. Am J Psychiatry 159:1112–1118, 2002

Fuchs E, Flugge G: Social stress in tree shrews: effects on physiology, brain function, and behavior of subordinate individuals. Pharmacol Biochem Behav 73:247–258, 2002

Gage FH: Mammalian neural stem cells. Science 287:1433–1438, 2000

Gilbertson MW, Shenton ME, Ciszewski A, et al: Smaller hippocampal volume predicts pathologic vulnerability to psychological trauma. Nat Neurosci 5:1242–1247, 2002

Gould E, Gross CG: Neurogenesis in adult mammals: some progress and problems. J Neurosci 22:619–623, 2002

Gould E, Beylin A, Tanapat P, et al: Learning enhances adult neurogenesis in the hippocampal formation. Nat Neurosci 2:260–265, 1999a

Gould E, Reeves AJ, Graziano MSA, et al: Neurogenesis in the neocortex of adult primates. Science 286:548–552, 1999b

Gould E, Vail N, Wagers M, et al: Adult-generated hippocampal and neocortical neurons in macaques have a transient existence. Proc Natl Acad Sci U S A 98:10910–10917, 2001

Halim ND, Weickert CS, McClintock BW, et al: Effects of chronic haloperidol and clozapine treatment on neurogenesis in the adult rat hippocampus. Neuropsychopharmacology 29:1063–1069, 2004

Harrison PJ: Neuropathology of primary mood disorder. Brain 125:1428–1449, 2002

Hirayasu Y, Shenton ME, Salisbury DF, et al: Subgenual cingulate cortex volume in first-episode psychosis. Am J Psychiatry 156:1091–1093, 1999

Ikonomidou C, Bosch F, Miksa M, et al: Blockade of NMDA receptors and apoptotic neurodegeneration in the developing brain. Science 283:70–74, 1999

Ikonomidou C, Bittigau P, Ishimaru MJ, et al: Ethanol-induced apoptotic neurodegeneration and the fetal alcohol syndrome. Science 287:1056–1060, 2000

Ikonomov OC, Manji HK: Molecular mechanisms underlying mood stabilization in manic-depressive illness: the phenotype challenge. Am J Psychiatry 156:1506–1514, 1999

Jacobs BL, van Praag H, Gage FH: Adult brain neurogenesis and psychiatry: a novel theory of depression. Mol Psychiatry 5:262–269, 2000

Jevtovic-Todorovic V, Hartman RE, Izumi Y, et al: Early exposure to common anesthetic agents causes widespread neurodegeneration in the developing rat brain and persistent learning deficits. J Neurosci 23:876–882, 2003

Kempermann G: Why new neurons? Possible functions for adult hippocampal neurogenesis. J Neurosci 22:635–638, 2002

Lemaire V, Koehl M, Le Moal M, et al: Prenatal stress produces learning deficits associated with an inhibition of neurogenesis in the hippocampus. Proc Natl Acad Sci U S A 97:11032–11037, 2000

MacQueen GM, Campbell S, McEwen BS, et al: Course of illness, hippocampal function, and hippocampal volume in major depression. Proc Natl Acad Sci U S A 100:1387–1392, 2003

Madsen TM, Treschow A, Bengzon J, et al: Increased neurogenesis in a model of electroconvulsive therapy. Biol Psychiatry 47:1043–1049, 2000

Malberg JE, Eisch AJ, Nestler EJ, et al: Chronic antidepressant treatment increases neurogenesis in adult rat hippocampus. J Neurosci 20:9104–9110, 2000

Manji HK, Moore GJ, Chen G: Lithium at 50: have the neuroprotective effects of this unique cation been overlooked? Biol Psychiatry 46:929–940, 1999

Manji HK, Moore GJ, Chen G: Clinical and preclinical evidence for the neurotrophic effects of mood stabilizers: implications for the pathophysiology and treatment of manic-depressive illness. Biol Psychiatry 48:740–754, 2000

Manji H, Drevets WC, Charney DS: The cellular neurobiology of depression. Nat Med 7:541–547, 2001

Mennerick S, Zorumski CF: Survival and neural activity in the developing nervous system. Mol Neurobiol 22:41–54, 2000

Mistry SK, Keefer EW, Cunningham BA, et al: Cultured rat hippocampal neural progenitors generate spontaneously active neural networks. Proc Natl Acad Sci U S A 99:1621–1626, 2002

Moore GJ, Bebchuk JM, Hasanat K, et al: Lithium increases N-acetyl-aspartate in the human brain: in vivo evidence in support of bcl-2's neurotrophic effects? Biol Psychiatry 48:1–8, 2000a

Moore GJ, Bebchuk JM, Wilds IB, et al: Lithium-induced increase in human brain grey matter. Lancet 356:1241–1242, 2000b

Moulder KL, Fu T, Melbostad H, et al: Ethanol-induced death of postnatal hippocampal neurons. Neurobiol Dis 10:396–409, 2002

Nakatomi H, Kuriu T, Okabe S, et al: Regeneration of hippocampal pyramidal neurons after ischemic brain injury by recruitment of endogenous neural progenitors. Cell 110:429–441, 2002

Öngür D, Drevets WC, Price JL: Glial reduction in the subgenual prefrontal cortex in mood disorders. Proc Natl Acad Sci U S A 95:13290–13295, 1998

Palmer TD, Schwartz PH, Taupin P, et al: Cell culture: progenitor cells from human brain after death. Nature 411:42–43, 2001

Rajkowska G: Postmortem studies in mood disorders indicate altered numbers of neurons and glial cells. Biol Psychiatry 48:766–777, 2000

Rajkowska G, Miguel-Hidalgo JJ, Wei J, et al: Morphometric evidence for neuronal and glial prefrontal cell pathology in major depression. Biol Psychiatry 45:1085–1098, 1999

Rajkowska G, Halaris A, Selemon LD: Reductions in neuronal and glial density characterize the dorsolateral prefrontal cortex in bipolar disorder. Biol Psychiatry 49:741–752, 2001

Rakic P: Neurogenesis in adult primate neocortex: an evaluation of the evidence. Nat Rev Neurosci 3:65–71, 2002

Santarelli L, Saxe M, Gross C, et al: Requirement of hippocampal neurogenesis for the behavioral effects of antidepressants. Science 301:805–809, 2003

Sapolsky RM: Glucocorticoids and hippocampal atrophy in neuropsychiatric disorders. Arch Gen Psychiatry 57:925–935, 2000

Schulman RG: Functional imaging studies: linking mind and basic neuroscience. Am J Psychiatry 158:11–20, 2001

Scott BW, Wojtowicz JM, Burnham WM: Neurogenesis in the dentate gyrus of the rat following electroconvulsive shock seizures. Exp Neurol 165:231–236, 2000

Seri B, Garcia-Verdugo JM, McEwen BS, et al: Astrocytes give rise to new neurons in adult mammalian hippocampus. J Neurosci 21:7153–7160, 2001

Shah PJ, Ebmeier KP, Glabus MF, et al: Cortical grey matter reductions associated with treatment-resistant chronic unipolar depression: controlled magnetic resonance imaging study. Br J Psychiatry 172:527–532, 1998

Shah PJ, Glabus MF, Goodwin GM, et al: Chronic, treatment-resistant depression and right fronto-striatal atrophy. Br J Psychiatry 180:434–440, 2002

Sheline Y, Wang P, Gado M, et al: Hippocampal atrophy in recurrent major depression. Proc Natl Acad Sci U S A 93:3908–3913, 1996

Sheline YI, Gado MH, Price JL: Amygdala core nuclei volumes are decreased in recurrent major depression. Neuroreport 9:2023–2028, 1998

Sheline Y, Sanghavi M, Mintun M, et al: Depression duration but not age predicts hippocampal volume loss in medically healthy women with recurrent major depression. J Neurosci 19:5034–5043, 1999

Sheline YI, Gado MH, Kraemer HC: Untreated depression and hippocampal volume loss. Am J Psychiatry 160:1516–1518, 2003

Shors TJ, Miesegaes G, Beylin A, et al: Neurogenesis in the adult is involved in the formation of trace memories. Nature 410:372–376, 2001

Song H, Stevens CF, Gage FH: Astroglia induce neurogenesis from adult neural stem cells. Nature 417:39–44, 2002a

Song H, Stevens CF, Gage FH: Neural stem cells from adult hippocampus develop essential properties of functional CNS neurons. Nat Neurosci 5:438–445, 2002b

Van Praag H, Christie BR, Sejnowski TJ, et al: Running enhances neurogenesis, learning, and long-term potentiation in mice. Proc Natl Acad Sci U S A 96: 13427–13431, 1999

Van Praag H, Schinder AF, Christie BR, et al: Functional neurogenesis in the adult hippocampus. Nature 415:1030–1034, 2002

Vythilingam M, Heim C, Newport J, et al: Childhood trauma associated with smaller hippocampal volume in women with major depression. Am J Psychiatry 159:2072–2080, 2002

Wang H-D, Dunnavant FD, Jarman T, et al: Effects of antipsychotic drugs on neurogenesis in the forebrain of the adult rat. Neuropsychopharmacology 29:1230–1238, 2004

Xu W, Cormier R, Fu T, et al: Slow death of postnatal hippocampal neurons by $GABA_A$ receptor overactivation. J Neurosci 20:3147–3156, 2000

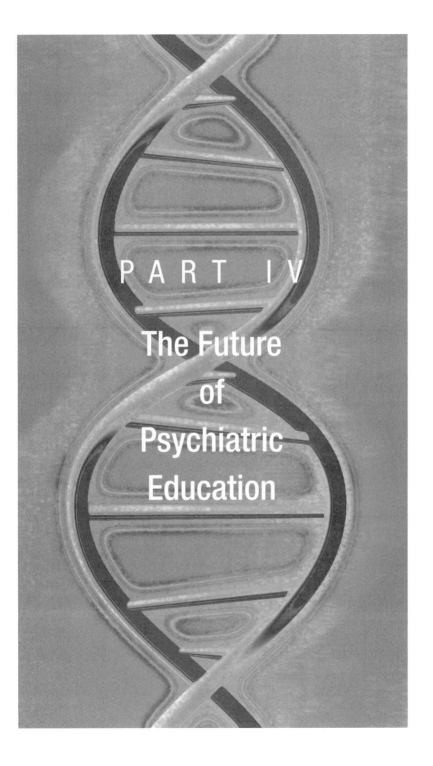

PART IV

The Future
of
Psychiatric
Education

Influence of Scientific Advances, Workforce Issues, and Educational Trends on Psychiatric Training

Eugene H. Rubin, M.D., Ph.D.

Charles F. Zorumski, M.D.

It is an extraordinary time in the evolution of psychiatry. Over the next 20 years, basic scientific advances are likely to lead to the development of more sophisticated treatments targeting specific disease mechanisms. During the same time span, the number of psychiatrists per 100,000 population will be substantially decreasing. Also, we are in the midst of a significant transition in medical education, namely a shift toward the evaluation of "competencies" in our trainees. Our goal in this chapter is to review these scientific, workforce, and educational trends and to discuss their impact on psychiatric education.

SCIENTIFIC ADVANCES

We are experiencing a neuroscientific and genetic revolution, which is generating results that are becoming increasingly clinically relevant.

The discovery of mechanisms underlying psychiatric symptoms and syndromes will promote the development of new diagnostic and therapeutic approaches. Advances in neuroimaging may lead to the ability to diagnose certain conditions at earlier stages, perhaps even allowing the detection of illness at a presymptomatic stage. Genetic epidemiologists are elucidating the complex relationships between genetic and environmental factors and psychiatric symptoms and syndromes. Advances in understanding the human response to stressors, including disasters or terrorist attacks, will help in the development of better treatments for trauma-related symptoms. Psychotherapy research is progressing and will likely lead to new and better therapies. Knowledge is expanding at such a rapid rate that it is important for educational leaders to identify areas that are essential for psychiatrists to fully master versus areas that are appropriate for psychiatrists to know well enough to foster collaboration with other mental health professionals.

Mechanisms of Illness

Dementia of the Alzheimer type (DAT) and narcolepsy provide instructive examples of how recent advances in our understanding of the pathophysiology of brain disorders can have direct relevance to psychiatrists. Although the first description of DAT was published in 1907 (Alzheimer 1907/1987), careful longitudinal studies to validate diagnostic criteria and elucidate the natural history of the illness were not conducted until the 1980s. About a decade later, families with rare, autosomal dominant subtypes of DAT began to be identified, and investigators were able to determine the specific genetic abnormalities associated with many of these familial forms. Models of the disease were produced in transgenic mice. Findings from these studies helped investigators formulate the amyloid cascade hypothesis, which relates the symptoms of the illness to the accumulation of excessive amounts of amyloid in the brain (Cummings 2004). Considerable evidence now supports this mechanism for DAT, and as a result, new treatments to slow the accumulation of amyloid or to enhance the clearance of accumulated amyloid are being investigated (Galasko et al. 2001; Wolfe 2002). These treatments may involve inhibitors of enzymes that form amyloid (secretase inhibitors) or antibodies that enhance the elimination of amyloid.

Psychiatrists treat patients with DAT, especially when symptoms such as agitation, psychosis, or depression are present. Families are often quite sophisticated in the questions they ask. Current information is available to them through the Alzheimer's Association as well as on the

Internet. Families may ask about the status of secretase inhibitor trials in DAT, the relationship of apolipoprotein E and DAT, or the use of antibodies in the diagnosis or treatment of DAT. Psychiatrists are expected to be up to date concerning such advances.

Currently, clinicians base the diagnosis of very mild DAT on information from interviews of the patient and a collateral source in order to determine whether significant changes involving memory and other cognitive functions are occurring. Examination of the patient and various test results are used to rule out other potential causes of the cognitive deterioration. Brain changes precede clinical symptoms by several years, however (Goldman et al. 2001), and methods of assessing such changes prior to the appearance of clinical symptoms are being developed. In vivo imaging of amyloid is one promising approach (Mathis et al. 2005). One can envision screening procedures for DAT parallel to mammography for breast cancer or colonoscopy for colon abnormalities. In addition to accurate detection of DAT, diagnostic methods based on disease mechanism should enable psychiatrists to differentiate, for example, very mild dementia with withdrawn behavior from depression with associated cognitive impairment. Psychiatrists will be expected to understand and utilize such diagnostic procedures.

Persons with Lewy body dementia may experience psychotic symptoms early in the course of the illness and may seek the aid of psychiatrists. The early symptoms of frontotemporal dementias, a third group of progressive dementias, may include marked personality changes, sometimes leading to psychiatric referral. Although less is known about the mechanisms of these dementias in comparison with DAT, Lewy body dementia involves abnormalities in a protein called *alpha synuclein* (see McKeith 2002), and certain frontotemporal dementias involve abnormalities in a protein called *tau* (Snowden et al. 2002). Within the next few decades, we are likely to have specific diagnostic techniques and mechanism-based treatments for these dementias as well.

Narcolepsy is another brain disorder with associated behavioral changes. Current, symptomatic treatments include stimulants and antidepressants. In recent years, great progress has been made in understanding the mechanisms underlying this illness (Krahn et al. 2001; Scammell 2003; Silber and Rye 2001). A polypeptide called *hypocretin* (also called *orexin*) has been identified and shown to be etiologically related to narcolepsy. Therapies based on hypocretin or hypocretin receptors may be developed (John et al. 2000). Many patients and their families know about these recent advances and expect their treating physicians to understand the latest findings. Although narcolepsy may not be an illness that many psychiatrists treat, the rate of progress in elucidating the mechanisms underlying this illness has been remarkable and demonstrates the potential for rapid, clinically relevant discoveries involving disorders of brain and behavior.

The mechanisms of an increasing number of neuropsychiatric illnesses are becoming better defined. It is only a matter of time before the pathophysiologies underlying some of the more traditional psychiatric disorders such as bipolar disorder, schizophrenia, or anorexia nervosa are discovered. Once such findings start to be reported, there will be a substantial increase in the number of basic science researchers investigating these areas, which in turn will enhance the rate of new findings.

Technology

New imaging procedures are providing better characterization of brain systems involved in specific psychiatric disorders. The detection of amyloid accumulation in patients with DAT may be possible in vivo (Mathis et al. 2005). Disease-related changes in the structure or function of regions such as the hippocampus, amygdala, prefrontal cortex, anterior cingulate, striatum, and thalamus are being characterized. Defining the functional neuroanatomy of systems underlying behavioral states and personality characteristics is feasible (Gusnard et al. 2001; Simpson et al. 2001). Targeting the delivery of highly specific medications to specific brain cells is no longer science fiction (Pardridge 2002). Such biomedical advances are exciting, and psychiatrists must have the appropriate background and training to understand and implement these advances.

Technological advances in genetics, including gene chip technology, will facilitate not only the discovery of specific genes and proteins involved in psychiatric disorders but also the determination of an individual's risk for certain disorders. With the use of gene chips, it will likely be possible to examine an individual's profile of genetic risk factors.

Treatments

Pharmacological Treatments

As disease mechanisms are elucidated, new pharmacotherapies will be developed based on these mechanisms. In addition, advances in pharmacogenetics may allow psychiatrists to select the most effective drugs for a particular individual based on the person's genetic profile (Evans and McLeod 2003; Kleyn and Vesell 1998). Similarly, a better understanding of the genetics of the cytochrome P450 system should improve the ability to minimize serious drug interactions (Cozza et al. 2003). As our understanding of character and temperament becomes more rigorous, the influence of personality characteristics on medication response will be clarified.

The population is aging. There are pharmacokinetic and pharmacodynamic differences in the handling of drugs by elderly patients. As people age, they also tend to take multiple medications. With the molecular and genetic revolution influencing drug development in all fields of medicine, there will be a tremendous increase in the number and classes of medications. As a result, the complexity of using psychiatric medications in the elderly and medically ill will increase.

As the relationship between genetic mechanisms and environmental factors is further clarified, the potential exists for targeting specific brain regions or cell types with pharmacotherapies or gene therapies (Pardridge 2002; Sapolsky 2003). With genetic techniques, it may be possible to design an intervention that would be triggered only under certain circumstances, such as highly stressful situations. Although such approaches are in their infancy, and there are myriad scientific and ethical issues to be resolved, such approaches are becoming increasingly feasible, and tomorrow's psychiatrist needs to understand the underlying scientific and ethical principles.

Psychotherapies

As new somatic treatments are developed, advances involving psychotherapies will also occur. The number of effective psychotherapies will likely increase. Mastering the administration of a specific psychotherapy is time intensive; however, nonphysician mental health professionals can be trained to safely and effectively administer specific psychotherapies, and it is likely that they will be increasingly involved in the delivery of formal psychotherapies. The need for nonphysician mental health professionals will grow for several reasons, including the demands of administering an increasing number of effective psychotherapies, an increased need for psychiatrists to devote their time to the biomedical advances, and the likelihood that there will be a substantial drop in the number of psychiatrists per 100,000 population (discussed later). Psychiatrists must become comfortable working with other members of the mental health team if they are to deliver care to all in need.

Other Treatments

As more is learned about the mechanisms underlying electroconvulsive therapies, new or improved approaches may be developed. Other treatment approaches are also under investigation, including magnetic therapies and chronic electrical stimulation. Implantation of brain stimulation devices to treat Parkinson's disease can be very effective, and it is possible that similar procedures will be discovered that help ameliorate refractory psychiatric symptoms. As discussed previously, genetic approaches to treatment are also likely.

DEMOGRAPHIC AND WORKFORCE ISSUES

As new and effective treatments are developed for psychiatric disorders, will there be sufficient numbers of psychiatrists to administer such treatments? Currently there is a need for more psychiatrists, but it will be difficult to increase the number in the foreseeable future. When the age distribution of psychiatrists is examined for the year 2002, it is evident that a larger percentage of psychiatrists are older in comparison with the rest of the physician population (Table 11–1). When this age distribution is examined over time (Figure 11–1) and the predicted growth of the U.S. population is also factored in, it seems clear that the number of psychiatrists per 100,000 will be decreasing substantially over the next two to three decades. This decrease will likely be in the range of 20%–25%.

A significant increase in the number of students entering psychiatric residencies would not be sufficient to counter this projected decrease. Furthermore, a rise in the number of psychiatry residents is unlikely to occur, because the federal government has set financial restrictions that effectively limit the total number of residency slots. Unless the government specifically mandates and funds more psychiatry positions or hospitals pay for positions from their own resources, the number of psychiatry residents will not increase.

TABLE 11–1.   Percentage of all physicians and psychiatrists in various age categories, 2002

	<35	35–44	45–54	55–64	≥65
All physicians ($N=853,187$)	16	25	25	16	18
Psychiatrists ($n=39,895$)	9	20	28	22	21

Source.   Data from Department of Physician Practice and Communications Information, Division of Survey and Data Resources: Physician Characteristics and Distribution, 2002–2004 Edition. Chicago, IL, American Medical Association, 2004.

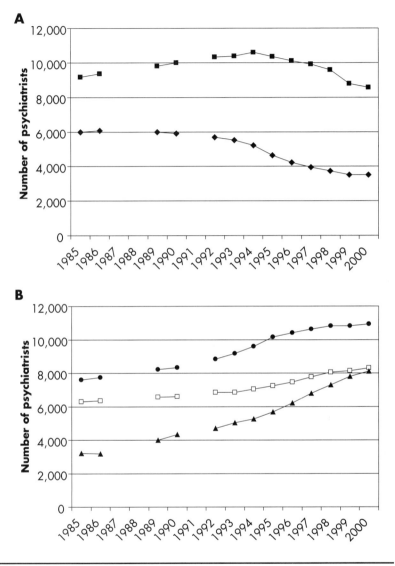

FIGURE 11–1.   Numbers of U.S. psychiatrists in various age groups over time.
(A) Psychiatrists younger than 45 years. *(B)* Psychiatrists 45 years and older.
Key (ages): ◆ < 35 years; ■ 35–44 years; ● 45–54 years; ❑ 55–64 years; ▲ ≥ 65 years.
Source.   Department of Physician Practice and Communications Information, Division of Survey and Data Resources: Physician Characteristics and Distribution, 2002–2003, 2001, 2000, 1999, 1997–1998, 1996–1997, 1995–1996, 1994, 1993, 1992, 1990, 1987, and 1986 Editions. Chicago, IL, American Medical Association.

[198]   PSYCHOPATHOLOGY IN THE GENOME AND NEUROSCIENCE ERA

There has been a recent increase in the number of American medical graduates choosing to specialize in psychiatry. At the present time, international medical graduates account for 40%–45% of psychiatry residents in the United States. A rise in the number of American medical school graduates selecting psychiatry most likely would not lead to an increase in the total number of residents but to a compensatory decrease in the number of international graduate trainees. Most international trainees practice in the United States after completion of their residency programs, and therefore, substituting American medical graduates for international medical graduates would not significantly influence the projected decrease in the workforce.

Although an increased number of American medical graduates entering psychiatry would not have a dramatic effect on the size of the workforce, it still would represent an important growth of interest in the field. The number of American medical graduates choosing psychiatry through the Resident Match has remained fairly constant at between 400 and 500 per year since the mid-1970s, with the exception of a transient increase to the mid 700s during the 1980s. In recent years, the number of American medical students choosing psychiatry through the Match gradually increased from the low 400s to over 650 in 2005. This rise in the number of American medical students interested in psychiatry may reflect increased general interest in the field, even in students who decide to train in other areas. It will become necessary for students interested in primary care disciplines to become comfortable with basic psychiatric diagnoses and treatments during their residencies, because they will need to recognize and manage uncomplicated psychiatric disorders.

EDUCATIONAL TRENDS

Currently, the most significant educational trend in graduate medical education is the movement toward the assessment of competencies. The Accreditation Council for Graduate Medical Education has recently instituted requirements for residency programs in all fields to evaluate the competency of residents in six areas: patient care, medical knowledge, practice-based learning and improvement, interpersonal and communication skills, professionalism, and systems-based practice (Accreditation Council of Graduate Medical Education 2001). These competency requirements compel programs to address both the science and the *art* of medicine—to evaluate not only biomedical skills but also psychosocial skills, including communication abilities, professionalism, and ethics.

In addition to the general competencies, the Residency Review Committee in psychiatry has implemented a set of psychiatry-specific competencies. These competencies involve five forms of psychotherapy: brief therapy, supportive therapy, cognitive-behavioral therapy, psychodynamic therapy, and combined psychotherapy and psychopharmacology (American Medical Association 2002). Although the current psychiatry-specific competencies may be meant to prevent psychiatrists from losing psychotherapeutic skills, it will become increasingly important that psychiatry-specific competency requirements not hinder residents from developing competence in essential biomedical skills in a rapidly evolving, biomedical world.

IMPLICATIONS FOR THE FUTURE OF PSYCHIATRIC EDUCATION

To summarize, there will be fewer psychiatrists per 100,000 population over the next several decades. Psychiatrists will be expected to be knowledgeable about clinically relevant biomedical advances, which will include progressive elucidation of genetic and biological mechanisms underlying many psychiatric disorders. As a result, diagnoses and treatments will become more complex. As the public becomes more aware of the disabilities that result from psychiatric disorders as well as the interaction of psychiatric with medical disorders, pressure to address the mental health needs of the population will grow.

In preparing for the future, it is essential that psychiatry residents have a strong background in the basic sciences—neurosciences, molecular sciences, cognitive sciences, pharmacology, epidemiology, and genetics—that will increasingly be the foundation of the field. Psychiatry residents also must acquire excellent communication skills and understand the process of various psychotherapies. In order to attend to the large number of patients in need of their unique expertise—that is, thorough, up-to-date knowledge of biomedical diagnostic and therapeutic approaches—psychiatrists will find it increasingly difficult to spend a large percentage of their work week administering time-intensive formal psychotherapies. Spending too little time with patients is also problematic, however. It takes significant time for a psychiatrist to gain an understanding of patients and their illnesses and for patients to develop a trusting relationship with the psychiatrist.

It will therefore become increasingly important for psychiatrists and nonphysician mental health professionals to coordinate their clinical efforts. Programs that train mental health professionals would benefit from increased communication and coordination. Understanding the unique as well as overlapping roles that physicians and various non-physician mental health professionals play can lead to a better matching of resources with needs.

The combination of a decreasing workforce of psychiatrists with increasingly effective treatments makes it important that primary care physicians learn the skills necessary to adequately manage patients with mild or stable psychiatric illness with minimal assistance from psychiatrists. Patients with common medical disorders such as heart disease and diabetes have comorbid psychiatric disorders, including significant depression. When depression is comorbid with such medical disorders, morbidity and mortality increase. Therefore, it is important for primary care physicians to be able to diagnose and treat both the medical and psychiatric disorders. In order to gain such skills, primary care residents should have greater exposure to psychiatry during their residency training, perhaps by participating in at least 1 month of a psychiatric inpatient or consultation rotation. In addition, senior psychiatry residents should be available routinely as consultants to primary care residency outpatient clinics in order to train primary care residents to recognize psychopathology in medically ill patients and to know when to treat and when to refer.

Besides covering the basic principles involved with the recognition, diagnosis, and treatment of psychiatric disorders, the psychiatric education of medical students should strive to develop an appreciation of the importance of psychiatry within the context of primary care medicine. Integration of psychiatric education throughout all 4 years of the curriculum will become increasingly important in this regard. An increase in the number of students entering the field would be helpful, but the increase would need to be substantial to reverse the downward trend in the number of psychiatrists per 100,000 population. It is important that medical students graduate with a positive attitude toward psychiatry so that they realize the importance of expanding their psychiatric knowledge and skills during primary care residencies. By combining the skills of the psychiatrists, nonphysician mental health professionals, and primary care physicians, we should be able to take full advantage of the extraordinary scientific advances and provide psychiatrically ill patients with effective treatments.

CONCLUSION

Biomedical advances are leading to mechanism-based treatments. These advances are likely to have a direct and profound influence on determining what will be expected of tomorrow's psychiatrists. Because of the biomedical nature of these advances, psychiatrists will be the mental health professionals with the medical training necessary to understand and implement these treatments. There will be fewer psychiatrists per 100,000 persons over the foreseeable future. This demographic trend will intensify the pressure on psychiatrists to deliver efficient and coordinated psychiatric care. Nonpsychiatric physicians will be needed to manage patients with stable psychiatric disorders. Various nonphysician mental health professionals will be essential in providing many services, including formal psychotherapies and coordinating psychosocial interventions. Anticipating these scientific and workforce trends should aid psychiatric educators in designing and implementing appropriate training for psychiatric residents, primary care residents, and medical students.

REFERENCES

Accreditation Council for Graduate Medical Education: General competencies, in Accreditation Council for Graduate Medical Education Outcome Project. Chicago, IL, Accreditation Council for Graduate Medical Education, 2001. Available at: http://www.acgme.org/outcome/comp/compFull.asp. Accessed February 13, 2003.

Alzheimer A: About a peculiar disease of the cerebral cortex (1907) (translated by Jarvik L, Greenson H). Alzheimer Dis Assoc Disord 1:7–8, 1987

American Medical Association: Program requirements for residency education in psychiatry, in Graduate Medical Education Directory 2002–2003. Chicago, IL, American Medical Association, 2002, pp 309–317

Cozza KL, Armstrong SC, Oesterheld JR: Concise Guide to Drug Interaction Principles for Medical Practice: Cytochrome P450s, UGTs, P-Glycoproteins, 2nd Edition. Washington, DC, American Psychiatric Publishing, 2003

Cummings JL: Alzheimer's disease. N Engl J Med 351:56–67, 2004

Department of Physician Practice and Communications Information, Division of Survey and Data Resources: Physician Characteristics and Distribution, 2002–2004 Edition. Chicago, IL, American Medical Association, 2004

Evans WE, McLeod HL: Pharmacogenomics: drug disposition, drug targets, and side effects. N Engl J Med 348:538–549, 2003

Galasko D: New approaches to diagnose and treat Alzheimer's disease: a glimpse of the future. Clin Geriatr Med 17:393–410, 2001

Goldman WP, Price JL, Storandt M, et al: Absence of cognitive impairment or decline in preclinical Alzheimer's disease. Neurology 56:361–367, 2001

Gusnard DA, Akbudak E, Shulman GL, et al: Medial prefrontal cortex and self-referential mental activity: relation to a default mode of brain function. Proc Natl Acad Sci U S A 98:4259–4264, 2001

John J, Wu MF, Siegel JM: Systemic administration of hypocretin-1 reduces cataplexy and normalizes sleep and waking durations in narcoleptic dogs. Sleep Res Online 3:23–28, 2000

Kleyn PW, Vesell ES: Genetic variation as a guide to drug development. Science 281:1820–1821, 1998

Krahn LE, Black JL, Silber MH: Narcolepsy: new understanding of irresistible sleep. Mayo Clin Proc 76:185–194, 2001

Mathis CA, Klunk WE, Price JC, et al: Imaging technology for neurodegenerative diseases: progress toward detection of specific pathologies. Arch Neurol 62:196–200, 2005

McKeith IG: Dementia with Lewy bodies. Br J Psychiatry 180:144–147, 2002

Pardridge WM: Drug and gene targeting to the brain with molecular Trojan horses. Nat Rev Drug Discov 1:131–139, 2002

Sapolsky RM: Gene therapy for psychiatric disorders. Am J Psychiatry 160:208–220, 2003

Scammell TE: The neurobiology, diagnosis, and treatment of narcolepsy. Ann Neurol 53:154–166, 2003

Silber MH, Rye DB: Solving the mysteries of narcolepsy: the hypocretin story. Neurology 56:1616–1618, 2001

Simpson JR Jr., Drevets WC, Snyder AZ, et al: Emotion-induced changes in human medial prefrontal cortex: II. during anticipatory anxiety. Proc Natl Acad Sci U S A 98:688–693, 2001

Snowden JS, Neary D, Mann DMA: Frontotemporal dementia. Br J Psychiatry 180:140–143, 2002

Wolfe MS: Therapeutic strategies for Alzheimer's disease. Nat Rev Drug Discov 1:859–866, 2002

CHAPTER 12

Crisis in American Psychiatric Education

*An Argument for the Inclusion of
Research Training for All Psychiatric Residents*

James J. Hudziak, M.D.

There are few things more humanitarian than the effective
use of knowledge to relieve suffering.

Samuel B. Guze 1970

There are not enough child psychiatrists in the United States, there are
not enough child psychiatrists pursuing research careers in the United
States, and there are not enough general psychiatrists pursuing research

---

The author has relied heavily on his experience on the Institute of Medicine
(IOM) Committee on Incorporating Research Into Psychiatry Residency Train-
ing. This committee was chaired by Thomas Boat, M.D., and directed by Michael
Abrams. See the IOM report (Institute of Medicine 2003) for a complete discus-
sion of the issues discussed in this chapter. The author wishes to thank Dr. Boat,
Mr. Abrams, and the 11 other committee members for their help.

careers in the United States. These three claims may seem debatable to those who are not aware of an emerging crisis in the lack of patient-oriented research in psychiatry; however, these claims are real (Institute of Medicine 2003) . Advances in neuroscience, psychiatric genetics, and treatment research in psychiatry have occurred at a tremendous rate over the past decade, making it likely that similar advances in diagnosis and therapeutics for psychiatric patients will be realized in the near future. As Fenton, James, and Insel (2004) point out,

> By any measure, research over the past two decades has yielded revolutionary leaps in understanding the human genome and how the brain functions, two areas of science fundamental to psychiatry. Recent discoveries have transformed our understanding of the brain, demonstrating how neurogenesis continues throughout adult life, mapping the dynamic nature of cortical connectivity that can change in response to experience, and identifying some of the categorical rules by which information is processed in the brain. Yet, during this same period, clinical psychiatry has remained relatively unchanged. (p. 263)

Perhaps at no other time in the history of psychiatry has there been so much public interest in our field. For reasons both good (the rapid advances in neuroimaging, behavioral sciences, and psychiatric genetics) and bad (recent reports of poorly studied or overprescribed medications), there has been a tremendous increase in the awareness of and interest in mental disorders. At a time when psychiatry, through careful patient-oriented research, has a chance to correct damaging misconceptions about psychopathology and psychiatric treatments, there is an insufficient number of well-trained child and adult research scientists to translate basic and clinical science discoveries into effective treatments. The only way to correct this shortage is to recruit, train, and retain more brilliant young scientific minds. Although such a process seems simple and forthright, many obstacles make it difficult to achieve this goal, including the failure of the psychiatry education infrastructure to generate the investigators necessary to make new discoveries and test new findings.

EVIDENCE OF THE PROBLEM

The burden of mental illness, the explosion of scientific and therapeutic discoveries (specifically in genetics and neuroscience) and the resulting increased social awareness of mental illness, and the relative absence of clinician-scientists to test new discoveries in patient-oriented research are the primary factors in the crisis facing psychiatry.

The Burden of Mental Illness

From a public health perspective, the burden of mental illness is often underestimated or even overlooked. Epidemiological data indicate that more than 450 million individuals suffer from a severe mental disorder (World Health Organization 2001). If suicide and substance abuse are combined with other psychopathologies, mental disease, in terms of disability-adjusted life years, is the number-one cause of morbidity and mortality (ahead of both cardiovascular disease and cancer). Given the prevalence of psychopathology and the morbidity and mortality associated with it, developing more effective ways to diminish the suffering associated with psychiatric illness should be a top priority for leaders around the world. Unfortunately, a disproportionately small amount of resources are devoted to this effort. In the face of such need, the call to "Do something!" can drown out the drive to do something better. If appropriate attention is given to addressing the burden of mental illness, and if new strategies for translating the new discoveries in genomics and neuroscience are forthcoming, there still must be practitioners who are ready to translate and implement new treatments as they emerge. Currently that is not the case.

Advances in Genetics and Neuroscience

For many years the brain was considered a black box; both clinicians and the general public accepted that uncovering the secrets of neuropathophysiology was unlikely. For as many years, genetic and environmental influences on human behavior were misunderstood, leading to a nature versus nurture debate in psychiatry. This situation led to misconceptions, partially perpetuated by psychiatry, and unfortunate divisions between the psychodynamic and biological branches of psychiatry.

We now know a great deal more about behavioral genetics and neuroscience than we did even a few years ago. With the recent advances in understanding the relative contributions of genetic and environmental influences, and their interactions, on common psychopathology has come a potential platform for all to agree. Rather than argue for a gene-only or environment-only perspective of etiopathogenesis, our new techniques allow us to test various nature–nurture hypotheses as they emerge. These techniques include a broad array of neuroscientific methods, such as positron-emission tomography (PET), functional magnetic resonance imaging (fMRI), and a variety of electroencephalographic approaches. It is not an overstatement to claim that neuropsychiatry finally has the goods to test its theories and to test hypotheses about causation. These approaches should lead directly to new understandings of psychopathology and to new treatments. However, while most psychiatrists now at least acknowledge the flaws in the dualistic view of mind and brain, the years of existing in parallel universes have made it difficult for scientists on both sides of the divide to reconcile their differences and build bridges necessary for successful integration.

Although few like to acknowledge the impact of this schism on recruitment and training, it remains a confound for extremists of both schools. It has been easy to portray psychoanalytic theories of etiology as silly, and proponents of the so-called biological school of psychiatry have been more than willing to do so over the past 30 years. However, it can be argued that the single-gene theories of the 1970s, 1980s, and early 1990s were equally silly. It is my opinion that psychiatry sits at a "tipping point" (Gladwell 2000) in its development. We are at a time when we must reconcile our differences as a field and move forward. Continued strife between the two so-called schools will continue to have catastrophic effects on our ability to recruit, train, and retain tough-minded psychiatrists.

Social Awareness and Misunderstanding of Mental Illness

It has become commonplace to see positron-emission tomography (PET) or functional magnetic resonance imaging (fMRI) images on the cover of *Time* or *Newsweek,* or reports on the major psychiatric disorders featured in the media. Equally common are reports of specific genetic and environmental influences on a variety of psychiatric illnesses. However, this increase in social awareness has come at a price. Nonpsychiatrist health care professionals, patients, and their families are all waiting—desperately—for "breakthroughs" in psychiatric treatment and prevention strategies. These discoveries have not been forthcoming in the way they have in other areas of medicine, and the public is beginning to become impatient. In terms of therapeutics, it is unfortunate that advances in specific psychiatric treatments over the past decade have lagged behind the explosion of new research findings. Although some advances in psychotherapies and pharmacotherapies have been realized, some of these advances have also been the focus of considerable criticism. Celebrities have taken up the debate, with passionate criticisms delivered on national television by movie stars such as Tom Cruise, wildly criticizing modern psychiatry and psychiatric treatments under his claim to be an "expert in the history of psychiatry" (*Good Morning America,* June 20, 2005), followed by a rebuttal from Brooke Shields, who has passionately described her battle with postpartum depression, in which she credits psychiatric care, both pharmacotherapeutics and psychotherapy, in the following ways: "But the drugs, along with weekly therapy sessions, are what saved me—and my family" and "If any good can come of Mr. Cruise's ridiculous rant, let's hope that it gives much-needed attention to a serious disease" (*New York Times,* "War of Words," July 1, 2005).

Mental illness is increasingly a topic with which our House and Senate members struggle. Representative Patrick Kennedy (D–Rhode Island) has authored and championed a bill in the House of Representatives, now being considered by the Senate, called The Child Healthcare Crisis Relief Act (H.R. 1106 and S. 537). To put it simply, this bill requests support to create incentives to help recruit and retain child mental health professionals providing direct clinical care and to improve, expand, or help create programs to train child mental health practitioners. This bill, along with the The Paul Wellstone Mental Health Parity Act (H.R. 1402) and The Keeping Families Together Act (H.R. 823 and S. 380), is an example of the positive momentum that has resulted from the increasing social awareness of psychopathology. While many political experts are pessimistic about the chances of these bills being enacted, the bills at least represent positive awareness. On the other hand, social negativism has also led to at least two bills (The Parental Consent Act [H.R. 181] and The Child Medication Safety Act [H.R. 1790]) proposed in Congress that are overtly hostile to the diagnoses and treatment of child psychiatric illness.

The Shortage of Psychiatric Researchers

It is difficult for many of us in psychiatric research to accept the mismatch between dramatic scientific advances and their practical application. Leaders in the psychiatric research and treatment communities have proposed that the lack of progress in prevention and therapeutics is due to the lack of physician-scientists who can translate basic science discoveries from genomics and neuroscience into new treatments. Michael Abrams and I, and the final IOM committee on training young psychiatrists, summarized the current situation in a report by the Institute of Medicine (IOM) (2003) entitled *Research Training in Psychiatry Residency: Strategies for Reform*:

> Great advances have been made in mental health care in recent years, and technological advances in the basic and clinical neural and behav-

ioral sciences offer considerable promise for future gains. At the same time, the burden of mental illness is very high, perhaps higher than any other single category of disease. Public knowledge of mental illness is increasing, as is public support for continued research. These realities should logically coincide with increasing involvement of psychiatrists in patient oriented research. (p. 23)

If we fail to repopulate the field of psychiatric research, realization of the gains of our neuroscience will be delayed even further.

A major factor that has led to the crisis in psychiatry is the drop in the number of young medical graduates who pursue training in psychiatry and, more specifically, psychiatric research. The number of new U.S. medical graduates entering psychiatry training dropped from 641 in 1991 to 524 in 2001, a decrease of 20% in just 10 years. Although that number has stabilized, at least for now, there remains a gap between a larger number of available training slots and interested candidates. Furthermore, the number of training positions authorized by the Committee on Graduate Medical Education has now been frozen. This unfortunate restriction may be due to institutional and programmatic prejudice against psychiatry. At the very least, there are financial obstacles, given the relative mismatch between revenue-generating activities that result from a psychiatric trainee's output versus the output of a surgical trainee. Whatever the explanation, even if a successful movement is generated to train more patient-oriented researchers in psychiatry, the corresponding cost will be a reduction in the number of candidates being trained to provide psychiatric patient care.

Dr. Steven Hyman, former director of the National Institute of Mental Health (NIMH) and strong advocate for patient-oriented researh in psychiatry, has argued that the absence of patient-oriented researchers in child psychiatry is already constraining the development of new, effective treatments in child psychiatry (Hyman 2002a). NIMH charged the IOM with studying what Dr. Hyman described as an alarming trend: Despite the increase in funding in mental health research over the past 10 years, the training of psychiatrist-researchers is not keeping pace with the needs of the patient-oriented mental health research (Institute of Medicine 2003, p. 5). Although there has been a general decline in the number of physician-researchers across medicine (Institute of Medicine 2003, p. 5), the trend is most alarming in psychiatry. Additionally, Dr. Hyman told the committee that he was alarmed by the apparently negative trends in the capacity of organized psychiatry to develop and test new technologies and that he and his program staff were particularly concerned about the limited expertise available in child psychiatry. He even suggested that child psychiatric research expertise was not sufficient to address efficacy and safety issues that have rapidly emerged regarding psychotropic medications frequently used in treating children. One survey of faculty at U.S. medical schools found that only 15% of academic psychiatrists spend more than half of their time engaged in research (Pincus et al. 1993). Another survey found that less than 2% of all U.S. psychiatrists consider research their primary activity (AAMC 2002). Moreover, the number of psychiatric graduates who complete research training fellowships dropped by 50% between 1992 and 2001, during the so-called Decade of the Brain (Fenton 2002; Hyman 2002b). There is evidence that the number of psychiatrists pursuing research fellowship training dropped nearly 40% (from 342 to 210 individuals) between 1992 and 2001 (American Psychiatric Association 2001). As Dr. Hyman (2002a) noted,

> Less than 10% of psychiatric residents express interest in academic or research careers upon entering training, and ultimately only a small fraction of these will pursue the rigors of an independent scientific career. The math is tragically straightforward: the number of psychiatrists who will be successfully engaged in science in the coming decades is approaching zero, this despite the incredible opportunities in our field.

MOTIVATION TO STUDY THE PROBLEM

Call for Study

The findings described in the preceding subsections spurred NIMH interest in the potential of a new approach to research training in psychiatric residencies. Because all psychiatrists are trained first as residents, the trend toward the disappearance of psychiatric research could perhaps be reversed by targeting the residency training period.

The reason for the shortages of adult and child psychiatric career investigators is multifactorial. Through careful study, it is clear that certain obstacles have impeded the recruiting, educating, and graduating of psychiatric clinicians who are prepared to engage in translational research. If we are to fulfill the promise of our field sparked by the previous "Decade of the Brain," we need to pursue a new roadmap laid out by the current director of the NIMH, Dr. Thomas Insel, in what he refers to as the "Decade of Translation," and populate our field with well-trained, effective, patient-oriented researchers in the areas of functional genomics, proteomics, and neuroscience. As Fenton, James, and Insel (2004) argue,

> The mission of the National Institute of Mental Health...is to reduce the burden of mental illness through research on mind, brain, and behavior. To achieve this mission, NIMH must ensure that two types of "translation" occur: 1) the translation of insights from neuroscience into better approaches to the diagnosis and treatment of psychiatric illness; and 2) the translation of what we have already learned about effective science-based treatment into the routine fabric of medical care delivery. An American public willing to invest tax dollars in biomedical research expects returns in the form of new treatments, effective strategies for prevention, and better health care. (p. 264)

As a result, the NIMH funded the work of the IOM.

The IOM Committee Charge

Michael Abrams and colleagues described the NIMH charge to the IOM as follows (Institute of Medicine 2003): The Committee on Incorporating Research into Psychiatry Residency Training was asked to review, among other issues, 1) current research training practices across typical and exemplary residency programs known for their devotion to research training; 2) the detailed training requirements mandated by the Residency Review Committees (RRCs) of the Accreditation Council for Graduate Medical Education (ACGME); and 3) the eligibility requirements for certification by the American Board of Psychiatry and Neurology (ABPN).

THE IOM REPORT

The final report of the Committee on Incorporating Research into Psychiatry Residency Training, *Research Training in Psychiatry Residency: Strategies for Reform* (Institute of Medicine 2003), was based on extensive literature reviews, consultations with a large array of outside experts, and informed deliberation. While focusing primarily on residency training, the career phase that constituted the committee's primary charge, the committee also touched on other critical tasks in career development, such as attracting research-oriented medical students to psychiatry and sustaining postresidency research interests and careers.

Recommendations

The IOM report provided an in-depth analysis of the obstacles to creating a research culture in psychiatry residency programs. Recommendations were broadly divided into five groups of recommendations (see Appendix 1):

1. Longitudinal factors (Figure 12–1).
2. The continuum of education (Figure 12–2)—the research and training milieu offered by individual residency programs. The curriculum, departmental and institutional facilities and finances, and ongoing research projects are all part of the training environment.
3. Regulatory issues: program accreditation and individual certification requirements that are governed by the Psychiatry RRC and that are under the auspices of the ACGME and the ABPN. Both the psychiatry RRC and the ABPN are independent, not-for-profit bodies that are largely run by volunteer psychiatrists.
4. Personal issues, including educational debt, family responsibilities, race/ethnicity, and gender, and clinical demands (service vs. training).
5. A final "overarching recommendation" aimed at creating an advisory or oversight council of stakeholders to ensure that the IOM recommendations were addressed.

The key stakeholders identified are the National Institutes of Health (NIH), American Psychiatric Association, the General Psychiatry and Child and Adolescent Psychiatry RRCs, ABPN, American Academy of Child and Adolescent Psychiatry, American Association of Chairmen of Departments of Psychiatry, American Association of Directors of Psychiatric Residency Training (AADPRT), and other professional psychiatric organizations and patient advocacy groups.

The IOM suggested that the NIMH should take the lead in organizing a national body, including major stakeholders (e.g., patient groups, department chairs) and representatives of organizations in psychiatry, that will foster the integration of research into psychiatric residency and monitor outcomes of efforts to do so. The IOM recommended that the group specifically collect and analyze relevant data, develop strategies to be put into practice, and measure the effectiveness of existing and novel approaches aimed at training patient-oriented researchers in psychiatry. The group should have direct consultative authority with the director of the NIMH and provide concise periodic reports to all interested stakeholders regarding its accomplishments and future goals.

Reaction to the Report

Numerous positive signs suggest that the IOM report is being considered in a serious way. Many efforts that were already under way (e.g., proposals for child psychiatry research training tracks both at local institu-

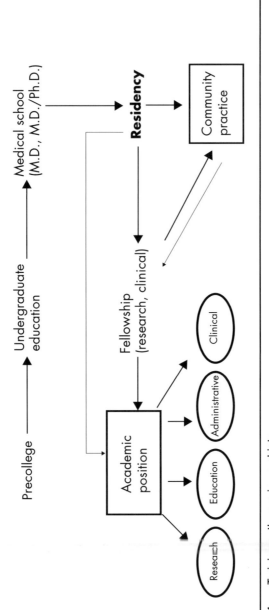

FIGURE 12–1.   Training pathways in psychiatry.

Source.   Institute of Medicine, Committee on Incorporating Research into Psychiatry Residency Training 2003.

Level[a]	Program components	Required department infrastructure
Solid research "track" (center of excellence)[b]	• 3 years core and 3 years research training • Strong connectivity between residency and postresidency research training • Residents aim for career (K) and a research (R) grant submission and a career in research • All components listed below	• Strong research culture/leadership • Expertise in several disciplines • Administrative support • Dedicated research resources • Research committee • Liaison with relevant facilities • Research training grants • Multiple major grants • Rich supply of mentors
Provision of research experience	• Coursework emphasizing methods and statistics • Longitudinal participation in a research project • Scholarly product • All components listed below	• Research culture • Research residency training director • Research funds • At least three major grants (e.g., RO1's) • Available mentors
Training of research-literate residents	• Coursework • Seminars • Grand rounds • Research rounds • Journal club • Visiting lectureships • Informatics[c]	• Minimal research • Few mentors

(Vertical arrow on left labeled "Continuum")

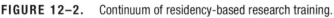

FIGURE 12–2. Continuum of residency-based research training.

[a]Most research-intensive program is listed at top. [b]Some information from David Kupfer interview in Meyer and McLaughlin 1998. [c]Knowledge about how to obtain, electronically archive, and efficiently review the latest in data germane to mental health research and practice.

Source. Adapted from Institute of Medicine 2003; reprinted from Meyer RE, McLaughlin CJ: "The Place of Research in the Mission of Academic Psychiatry," in *Between Mind, Brain, and Managed Care: The Now and Future World of Academic Psychiatry.* Edited by Meyer RE, McLaughlin CJ. Washington, DC, American Psychiatric Press, 1998, pp. 77–96. Used with permission.

tions [e.g., Yale Child Study Center] and supported by the American Academy of Child and Adolescent Psychiatry) have been energized. Perhaps the most profound response has come from the NIMH itself with the creation of the National Psychiatry Training Council (NPTC). This group of experts was created by NIMH Director Dr. Thomas Insel in response to the recommendation from the IOM that there be established a "national coordinating body to foster the integration of research training into psychiatry residency and to monitor the outcome of efforts to do so." Dr. Insel charged a group of stakeholders with the following (as reported in American Psychiatric Association 2004):

- "Develop a detailed vision for reform of psychiatric residency training that includes more flexible core training requirements designed to ensure clinical competency while fostering earlier specialization and in-depth training for areas such as patient-oriented research, geriatric psychiatry, and public psychiatry."
- "Identify steps to be undertaken by each stakeholder organization independently and by *all* key stakeholders working together in partnership."
- "Develop plans and timelines for accomplishing the change."

The task force comprises up to nine groups covering the main areas of influence: Model Programs, Pipeline (Recruitment), Mentorship, Research Literacy, Regulatory Revisions, Retention, Funding/Finances, Outcomes, and Dissemination (for a list of the chairs of each groups, see American Psychiatric Association 2004). The groups were charged to "propose recommendations that will define the psychiatrist of 2010 or 2020, but that are truly feasible [to implement] within that timeline; to think boldly, with both eyes on implementation; and to put forth specific, step-by-step, action-oriented proposals while emphasizing the necessary integration of activities across the groups." It is the goal of the NPTC to advocate for and lead the field of psychiatry to influence key regulatory groups, such as the RRCs, as soon as the fall of 2005, in preparation for defining the necessary skills for psychiatry residency research training of future psychiatrists.

The NPTC has established a group of action-oriented, implementation-focused task forces. Each task force is charged with compiling creative, future-oriented, and, most important, feasible recommendations with measurable outcomes for implementation within the next 5–10 years. Task force membership, comprising more than 90 leading psychiatrists, includes but is not limited to members of the NPTC. Many others are also being asked to participate, based on specific areas of expertise and stakeholder membership. Each task force is expected to "cross-talk" and integrate its ideas and recommendations. In this way, each recommendation will have to be considered in relation to regulatory modifications that might involve the National Institutes of Health (NIH), ACGME, ABPN, and/or other institutions and agencies, each of which has to be considered in relation to each recommendation (i.e., "impact statements"). Task force recommendations are expected to be as explicit as possible, with each recommendation designating the exact steps that various stakeholder groups will be expected to implement if improvements are to occur.

On the basis of the IOM recommendations, some of the stakeholder groups are already moving ahead. The American Psychiatric Association appointed Charles F. Reynolds III, M.D., Professor of Psychiatry, Neurology, and Neuroscience at the University of Pittsburgh School of Medicine, to the RRC for General Psychiatry, and myself to the RRC for Child and Adolescent Psychiatry. As an indication that the IOM's emphasis on research training during psychiatric residency training is being seriously considered, Michael H. Ebert, M.D., Chair of the RRC, has already made plans for the group to consider proposals from residency programs to incorporate more flexible programming that may foster psychiatric research training during residency for select individuals (e.g., the innovative child and adolescent programs developed by Leckman's group at Yale Child Study Center). Many additional innovative suggestions are expected to emerge.

The AACDP endorsed the anticipated IOM recommendations during a meeting held in Washington, D.C., in November 2003 and attended by most of the key stakeholders, and it recently held another retreat planning meeting in Sonoma in July 2004 to sustain momentum. This meeting was attended by Dr. Insel and representative leaders of other relevant NIH institutes and the Substance Abuse and Mental Health Services Administration (SAMHSA), AADPRT representatives, and medical student educators.

CONCLUSION

The work of the IOM presaged the ongoing work of the National Psychiatry Training Council, the Accreditation Council on Graduate Medical Education Residency Review Committees, and the American Board of Psychiatry and Neurology. Each of these groups is working toward the goal of improving the way psychiatry residents are recruited, trained, and retained, with the long-term goal of taking advantage of the advances in our field. Perhaps by integrating genetics and neuroscience with public health, epidemiology, and child development in teaching programs, we can attract more students and produce more scientifically minded physicians. We must do this while simultaneously emphasizing the remarkable advances in evidence-based psychotherapies. We can end dualistic fallacies by showing that our new techniques provide evidence for the mechanisms of action for both pharmacological and talk, cognitive, and behavioral therapies.

If we, as stakeholders, do not seriously address the crisis in both medical student and resident education in psychiatry, we risk putting ourselves in the unenviable position of discovering new ways to help our patients but not having the person-power to do so. We must produce new scientists in basic, applied, and patient-oriented research endeavors.

Finally, although it is clear that most great genomic and neuroscience researchers are not psychiatrists, we must train new psychiatrists in research principles. As we seek to achieve this goal through careful education of students at all ages by debunking the damaging misconceptions about psychopathology by bridging the gap between neuroscience, neuropsychiatric genetics, and public perception, we must start with our residents. By training all residents in these principles, we prepare them to practice psychiatry in this new era, introduce them to the possibilities of research careers, and, perhaps most importantly, train them as ambassadors of our field.

REFERENCES

American Psychiatric Association: Research Fellowship Directory: Online Directory of Research Fellowship Opportunities. 2001. Available at: http://www.psych.org/research/APIRE/fellow71601.cfm. Accessed May 30, 2005.

American Psychiatric Association: Psychiatric Research Report: Summer 2004. Available at: http://www.psych.org/research/dor/prr/prr-summer 2004.pdf. Accessed May 31, 2005.

Association of American Medical Colleges: AAMC Data Book: Statistical Information Related to Medical Education. Washington, DC, Association of American Medical Colleges, 2002

Fenton WS: Sponsor presentation of study genesis and charge presentation at the Institute of Medicine Committee on Incorporating Research Into Psychiatry Residency Training. Washington, DC, April 12, 2002

Fenton WS, James R, Insel T: Commentary on "Psychiatry Residency Training, the Physician-Scientist, and the Future of Psychiatry" by Yager et al. Academic Psychiatry 28:263–266, 2004

Gladwell M: The Tipping Point: How Little Things Can Make a Big Difference. New York, Little, Brown, 2000

Hyman SE: Integrating neuroscience, behavioral science, and genetics in model psychiatry, in Modern Psychiatry: Challenges in Educating Health Professionals to Meet New Needs. A Conference Sponsored by the Josiah Macy Jr Foundation. Edited by Hager M. New York, Josiah Macy Jr Foundation, 2002a

Hyman SE: Obstacles to residency-based research training in psychiatry. Presentation at the Institute of Medicine Committee on Incorporating Research Into Psychiatry Residency Training. Washington, DC, June 18, 2002b

Institute of Medicine: Careers in Clinical Research: Obstacles and Opportunities. Washington, DC, National Academies Press, 1994

Institute of Medicine: Clinical Research Roundtable: Summary of the June 2000 Meeting of the Clinical Research Roundtable. Washington, DC, National Academies Press, 2000

Institute of Medicine, Committee on Incorporating Research into Psychiatry Residency Training: Research Training in Psychiatry Residency: Strategies for Reform. Washington, DC, National Academies Press, 2003. Available at: http://www.nap.edu/catalog/10823.html. Accessed April 26, 2005.

Pincus HA, Dial TH, Haviland MG: Research activities of full-time faculty in academic departments of psychiatry. Arch Gen Psychiatry 50:657–664, 1993

U.S. Department of Health and Human Services: Report of the Surgeon General's Conference on Children's Mental Health: A National Action Agenda. Washington, DC, U.S. Department of Health and Human Services, 2000

World Health Organization: The World Health Organization Report 2001: Mental Health: New Understanding, New Hope. Geneva, World Health Organization, 2001

APPENDIX 1: IOM SUMMARY OF OBSTACLES IN RESEARCH TRAINING AND RECOMMENDATIONS FOR INTERVENTION[1]

Longitudinal Factors

• **Obstacle:** Research opportunities are fragmented across the multiple levels and years of training.
  Recommendation: Departments of psychiatry should organize optional research experiences and mandatory research didactics in res-

---

[1]Reprinted with permission from Yager J, Greden J, Abrams M, et al.: "The Institute of Medicine's Report on Research Training in Psychiatry Residency: Strategies for Reform—Background, Results, and Follow Up." *Academic Psychiatry* 28:267–274, 2004.

idency as early steps in research career development pathways, leading from residency to a junior faculty appointment. Federal and private
agencies should expand mechanisms that encourage psychiatry trainees to enter research careers and move, without interruption, from
residency to a research fellowship to a faculty position designed to promote independence as a patient-oriented investigator.

Institutional Factors

- **Obstacle:** Clinical requirements are excessive and prevent tailored
  training.
  Recommendation: The ABPN and the RRC should make the requirements for board certification and residency accreditation more flexible so research training can occur during residency at a level that
  significantly increases the probability of more residents choosing research as a career. The committee further recommends that residents
  who successfully fulfill core requirements at an accelerated pace,
  with competency being used as the measure, be allowed to spend the
  time thus made available to pursue research training.
- **Obstacle:** Many training programs lack research education components.
  Recommendation: The ABPN and the RRC should require patient-
  oriented research literacy as a core competency of residency training
  in adult and child and adolescent psychiatry. Program directors and
  the ABPN should evaluate residents on these competencies.
- **Obstacle:** Researchers are not sufficiently involved in setting expectations for training curricula and achievement of competencies.
  Recommendation: The organizations that nominate members for the
  Psychiatry RRC and the ABPN should include on their nomination
  lists substantial numbers of extramurally funded, experienced psy-
  chiatrist-investigators who conduct patient-oriented research.
- **Obstacle:** Despite obvious major advances in both neuroscience and
  the behavioral sciences, resources to support research training are
  limited; stigma works against optimal mental health care funding.
  Recommendation: The broad psychiatry community should work
  more aggressively to encourage university presidents, deans, and hospital chief executive officers to give greater priority to the advance-
  ment of mental health through investments in leadership, faculty,
  and infrastructure for research and research training in psychiatry departments.

- **Obstacle:** Researchers often are not involved in direct resident training.
  Recommendation: Academic institutions and their psychiatry residency training programs should reward the involvement of patient-oriented research faculty in the residency training process. The NIMH should take the lead in identifying funding mechanisms to support such incentives.
- **Obstacle:** Curricula are needed that incorporate research training across the range and time constraints of residency programs.
  Recommendation: The NIMH, foundations, and other funding agencies should provide resources to support efforts to create competency-based curricula for research literacy and more comprehensive research training in psychiatry that are applicable across the spectrum of adult (general) and child and adolescent residency training programs. Supported curriculum development efforts should include plans for educating faculty to deliver each new curriculum, as well as plans for evaluating each curriculum's success in training individuals to competency and in recruiting and training successful researchers.
- **Obstacle:** Resources to move programs to the next level of research training are scarce, especially for small or modest-sized programs.
  Recommendation: The NIMH should support those departments that are poised to improve their residency-based research training to achieve measurable increases in patient-oriented research careers among their trainees. Support should include funds to

  - Hire faculty and staff dedicated to research and research training efforts.
  - Acquire equipment and enhance facilities for research training.
  - Initiate pilot and/or short-term research activities for residents.
  - Educate adult and child and adolescent residency training directors and other faculty in how to promote and guide research career planning. This recommendation acknowledges that talented researchers emerge from programs of all sizes, not just from large ones that are currently funded most heavily with research grants.

Personal Factors

- **Obstacle:** Education debt and low compensation deter the choice of a research career.
  Recommendation: The NIMH and other funding agencies should seek mechanisms to offer increased financial incentives, such as loan repayment, to trainees who commit to research training and research involvement beyond core psychiatry residency.

- **Obstacle:** Trainees have pessimistic views of research careers and can be uninformed about research opportunities.
  Recommendation: Individuals and institutions involved in the education and mentoring of medical students, residents, and fellows should strongly convey to these trainees the benefits (professional and societal) associated with patient-oriented research in psychiatry. Promotion strategies might include support for student interest groups; brochures, websites, and other media; and summer research training opportunities.
- **Obstacle:** Talents are underutilized (the following three recommendations address this issue).
  Recommendation: Departments of psychiatry supported by the NIMH and other psychiatric organizations should provide leadership in recruiting and retaining more women for psychiatry research careers. Such efforts should include

  - Increasing part-time training and job sharing opportunities.
  - Developing a critical mass of female role models and mentors.
  - Working with institutions to improve child day care programs.
  - Addressing institutional promotion and tenure issues, such as the tenure clock, that may be perceived as barriers to female trainees.
  - Educating women about the time flexibility of research careers.

  Recommendation: Psychiatry training programs, academic medical centers, psychiatry organizations, and the federal government should work together to facilitate research training for international medical graduates who have the potential to make outstanding research contributions to psychiatry. Retention of the most productive of these IMGs in U.S. academic psychiatry programs should also be a joint effort.
  Recommendation: Psychiatric research training programs should increase the numbers of underrepresented minority researchers in their training programs by employing the following strategies:

  - Recruit minority faculty in multiple disciplines to serve as role models and mentors.
  - Pursue funding from NIMH and other funding agencies that support minorities.
  - Inform more minority psychiatrists about research training and funding opportunities.

Overarching Recommendation

- **Obstacle:** Monitoring data are lacking, and there is no centralized plan for research training.

  Recommendation: The NIMH should take the lead in organizing a national body, including major stakeholders (e.g., patient groups, department chairs) and representatives of organizations in psychiatry, that will foster the integration of research into psychiatric residency and monitor outcomes of efforts to do so. This group should specifically

  - Collect and analyze relevant data.
  - Develop strategies to be put into practice.
  - Measure the effectiveness of existing and novel approaches aimed at training patient-oriented researchers in psychiatry. The group should have direct consultative authority with the director of the NIMH, and also should provide concise periodic reports to all interested stakeholders regarding its accomplishments and future goals.

APPENDIX 2: NATIONAL PSYCHIATRY TRAINING COUNCIL TASK FORCES AND CHARGES[2]

Model Programs

- Review programs from other disciplines (internal medicine, triple-board, neurology M.D./Ph.D., etc.) and from the IOM report to benefit from their experiences and reviews. Consider pros and cons of "non-traditional" models, e.g., M.D./Ph.D., Masters/Ph.D., and Ph.D. or Masters in combination with residency.
- Identify and summarize key elements of key model programs regardless of academic focus.
- Recommend steps for different departments to determine whether they should focus on one type of model (e.g., residency research track, clinical investigator track, clinical educator track, M.D./Ph.D./residency, etc.) or seek to achieve a balance of several programs.

---

[2]Reprinted with permission from Yager J, Greden J, Abrams M, et al.: "The Institute of Medicine's Report on Research Training in Psychiatry Residency: Strategies for Reform—Background, Results, and Follow Up." *Academic Psychiatry* 28:267–274, 2004.

What resources are required for a department to sustain an entire portfolio of model programs? Emphasize importance of creating residency programs that are flexible (i.e., all programs do not need to look the same).

- Focus on training models for clinical investigations and building interdisciplinary teams for translational work.
- Establish procedures to catalyze submission of three or four programs that will meet NPTC goals, generate support from key stakeholder organizations, and are likely to meet RRC approval. Estimate annual resources (e.g., financial, time, mentoring) for different model programs, and types of departments in which models might be possible.
- Emphasize pursuit of competencies that are not solely time-linked and strategies for attaining these competencies.
- Recommend required steps for other task forces and key stakeholders if model programs are to be sustained.
- Recommend how IT (Information Technology) advances may help future educational research training.

Pipeline (Recruitment)

- Set annual goals, objectives, and metrics for increasing the flow into clinical/translational academic activities. The APA Council on Research set a target of "doubling the number of psychiatrist investigators by 2010." Is that still appropriate?
- Promote involvement with and leadership of medical student psychiatry education directors.
- Identify career pipeline "turning points" where we might lose potential clinical researchers and formulate strategies to respond at these turning points.
- Recommend and catalyze appropriate groups to develop packages to assist local recruitment programs for high school, undergraduate and medical students.
- Suggest mechanisms to enable students at lower levels to become involved in research projects that lead to scientific publications.
- Suggest innovative strategies to more successfully convey the excitement of neurosciences, behavioral sciences, and clinical research to target populations.

Mentorship

- Set performance standards for what constitutes a successful mentor, and seek to publish this in a national journal.
- Assist chairs of departments in enhancing the pool of mentors (e.g., designated appointments as "mentor," protected time, incentives for funded grants, NARSAD [National Alliance for Research on Schizophrenia and Depression] awards, etc).
- Suggest strategies to deal with fiscal barriers, mentorship as requirement for promotion, linking recruitment to mentorship.
- Review feasibility of "mentorship tracks" for talented faculty.
- Recommend steps for training mentors, especially those who might work in clinical and translational arenas (e.g., national meetings, R-25 grants, NIMH/National Institute on Drug Abuse [NIDA]/National Institute on Alcohol Abuse and Alcoholism [NIAAA] conferences).

Research Literacy

- Review state-of-the-art literature on accepted principles of evidence-based medicine.
- Recommend strategies for chairs, training directors, RRC, etc., to adapt core principles to psychiatry residency education.
- Develop innovative strategies for requiring and achieving research literacy for all residents, not just those aiming for an academic career.
- Review and recommend steps for chairs and training directors to understand the considerable current flexibility within RRC guidelines to improve research literacy education among residents.
- Recommend strategies and identify implementation stakeholders responsible for incorporating educational steps designed to achieve research literacy into new model programs.
- Recommend strategies and identify implementation stakeholders responsible for measuring performance and outcome assessments.
- Formulate strategies to improve skills and training for AADPRT members and residency education directors to lead their local research literacy efforts.

Regulatory Revisions

- Work closely with Model Programs Task Force to ensure that key stakeholders (e.g., AACDP and AADPRT) jointly submit several feasible and effective proposals to RRC.

- Review and recommend steps for chairs and training directors to obtain greater understanding about the current flexibility within RRC guidelines so that research literacy and training of clinical/translational investigators can be improved instantly.
- Identify optimal targets for regulatory revisions that will enhance flexibility (e.g., reduction or change of time-based competency requirements).
- Develop strategies and work with the Dissemination Task Force to actively and effectively communicate any changes that RRC approves to the field, including dissemination to institute directors, deans, chairs, hospital directors, and medical students.
- Work in partnership with leadership of the American Board of Psychiatry and Neurology (ABPN) to ensure synergy and acceptance of all emerging regulatory revisions.
- Coordinate a meeting with ACGME that involves NPTC leadership, AADPRT, AACDP, and RRC to review and catalyze this process.

Retention

- Outline barriers and variables, develop retention strategies, and pick a few key strategies that the committee can address.
- Recommend new and innovative strategies to improve mechanisms that help overcome existing barriers, e.g., debt relief (by identifying new sources of support), and modifications of training grants to permit such relief.
- Involve industry, foundations; seek other philanthropy initiatives.
- Recommend different strategies for different departments and academic programs, depending upon their resources and their targets.
- Develop more nuanced and successful exit strategies for seamless and smooth transitions for those who do not succeed in academic investigations (since not all who attempt research will prove to be suitable).
- Develop methods to communicate strategies for effective retention, including provision of specific guidelines about how key stakeholder groups should consider applying them.
- Work closely with Outcomes and Mentorship Task Forces to measure impact of new programs on retention.

Funding/Finances

- Determine estimates of expenses for new research training initiatives for departments, hospitals, NIH Institutes, and others.

- Set annual goals, objectives, metrics, and financial targets to help meet expenses that will be required for the annual increase in numbers of investigators.
- Recommend strategies for each key stakeholder group to tackle, independently and in concert with others, to help meet these annual goals.
- Work with foundations to enhance their involvement in this important objective.
- Suggest new strategies to enhance training of mentors and how such initiatives might be funded during the time period when departments and NIH Institutes are struggling with financial constraints.
- Recommend strategies to involve the Veterans Administration [Veterans Affairs] healthcare system and to fund research training programs that emphasize interdisciplinary and translational initiative that are supportive of the NIH Roadmap.

Outcomes

- Define parameters of success and check these with respective Task Forces.
- Identify a core set of "vital signs" that can be tracked over time.
- Develop and implement measurement processes that are cost-efficient and applicable to existing databases, and that work across all key stakeholder groups (NIMH, NIAAA, NIDA, VA, SAMHSA, Chairs, training directors, etc.).
- Evaluate outcome from programs that have already been implemented in other specialties; e.g., internal medicine "short track" versus traditional model, Triple Board model, M.D./Ph.D., etc.
- Develop strategies for dealing with the confound of self-selection into a particular type of program.
- Develop a simple, understandable method for reporting summary progress in each of the key arenas, e.g., model program implementation (B–, Pipeline/Recruitment, C, Retention, A–, Regulatory Revisions, etc.).
- Compare the relative impact of one model program vs. others.
- Recognize that while the majority of work of this Task Force may occur at a later time, the parameters of outcome monitoring should be developed early and iteratively improved via interactions with respective Task Forces.

Dissemination

- Work with overall NPTC, NIH leaders, and leaders of key stake-holder organizations to summarize and disseminate the rationale, goals, and strategies to further broaden the base of support.
- Lead preparation and publication of progress reports in leading journals in the field, including those that are influential in shaping regulatory and fiscal policies.
- Involve each NPTC Task Force in dissemination of its products.
- Retain contact with and provide feedback to IOM Committee members to gain from their expertise.
- Arrange for speakers to present at major national stakeholder meetings.
- Work with Outcomes Task Force to arrange venues for dissemination to major meetings on an annual basis (e.g., ACNP, APA, AADPRT meeting).
- Disseminate periodic updates to APA members, Chairs, AADPRT members, etc., using the APA listserv, available web sites, and other effective and cost-efficient venues.

APPENDIX 3: COMMENTARY ON "PSYCHIATRY RESIDENCY TRAINING, THE PHYSICIAN-SCIENTIST, AND THE FUTURE OF PSYCHIATRY" BY YAGER ET AL.[3]

By Wayne Fenton, M.D., Regina James, M.D., and Thomas Insel, M.D.

In response to this overarching recommendation, the director of NIMH established the National Psychiatry Training Council (NPTC) under the co-leadership of John Greden, M.D., from the University of Michigan and James Leckman, M.D., from the Yale Child Study Center, an adult academic psychiatrist and a child and adolescent academic psychiatrist, respectively. Conceived as a body with an initial 2-year charter, the NPTC's initial charges are

---

[3]*Academic Psychiatry* 28:263–266, 2004. Commentary on Yager J, Greden J, Abrams M, et al.: "The Institute of Medicine's Report on Research Training in Psychiatry Residency: Strategies for Reform—Background, Results, and Follow Up." *Academic Psychiatry* 28:267–274, 2004. Reprinted with permission.

- Develop a detailed vision for reform of psychiatric residency training that includes more flexible core training requirements designed to ensure clinical competency while fostering earlier specialization and in-depth training in areas such as patient-oriented research, geriatric, and public psychiatry.
- Identify steps to be undertaken by each stakeholder organization independently and by all key stakeholders working together in partnership to actualize this vision.
- Develop plans and timelines for accomplishing these steps.

Key stakeholder organizations were identified...and [they] nominated one or more members to serve on the training council. Collectively, these are the organizations that define the structure and content of psychiatric education in the United States. We are hopeful that, convened together for the first time with a clear charge and commonality of purpose, they will achieve reforms to meaningfully enhance not only patient-oriented research training opportunities but also training in other areas where critical manpower shortages exist such as public sector, child and adolescent psychiatry, and geriatric psychiatry. The NPTC initially met on April 7, 2004, in Bethesda, Maryland, to organize an approach to setting goals and initiating the process of reform. To date, a number of task forces have been formed to address both the Council's specific charge and related issues, including model programs, pipeline, regulatory revisions, mentorship, research literacy, retention, finance, outcomes, and dissemination.

From the NIMH vantage point, two central concepts should guide the reform of psychiatric residency training: 1) flexibility to permit specialization and 2) grounding in the principles of evidence-based medicine.

A major criticism of evidence-based practice is that it ignores intuition, experience, and clinical judgment; deemphasizes the importance of the physician-patient relationship; and renders the practice of medicine sterile and formulaic. Contrary to these criticisms, most proponents of evidence-based practice agree "that a cookbook is not a cook." Aspects of the "art of medicine" can only be derived from the opinions and experience of exceptional clinicians who have a gift for precise observation, careful diagnosis, and excellent judgment in making complex clinical management decisions. Evidence-based reviews of treatment effectiveness increasingly suggest that for the most severe disorders such as schizophrenia, integrated psychosocial and biological treatments yield superior outcomes. The psychiatrist's understanding of human behavior and human experience, derived both from didactic study and supervised clinical work, should place him or her in the unique position of being able to create and monitor treatment plans that integrate both biological and psychosocial perspectives.

The time is now right for a rethinking and reform of psychiatric residency training. The IOM report, convening of the National Psychiatry Training Council, and unprecedented cooperation of diverse stakeholders create what may be a once-in-a-generation opportunity to achieve meaningful change. The future of psychiatry as a medical specialty depends critically on our success in training physician-scientists to translate advances in neuroscience into new treatments and cures and research-literate clinicians who can ensure that patients receive the best science-based care.

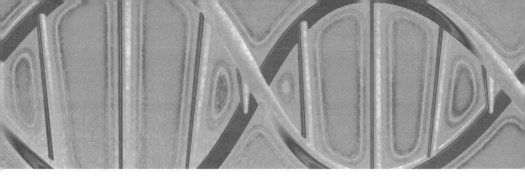

Index

Page numbers printed in **boldface** type refer to tables or figures.